THE FOUR PILLAR PLAN

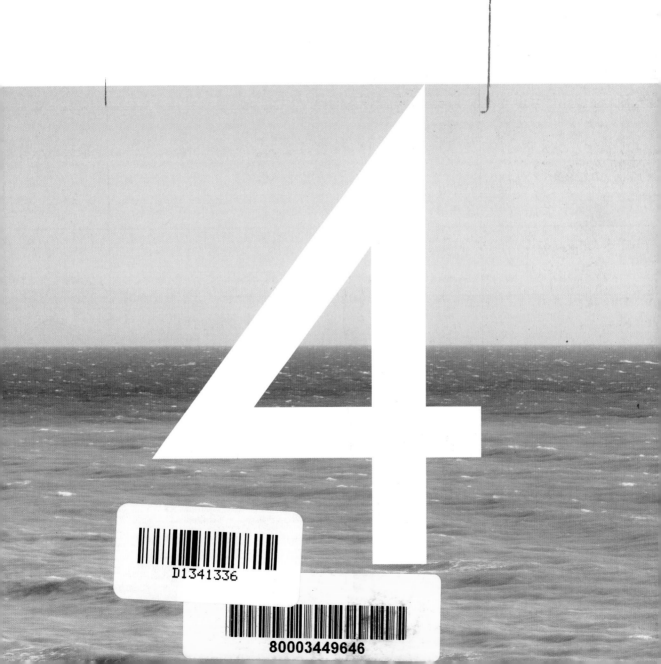

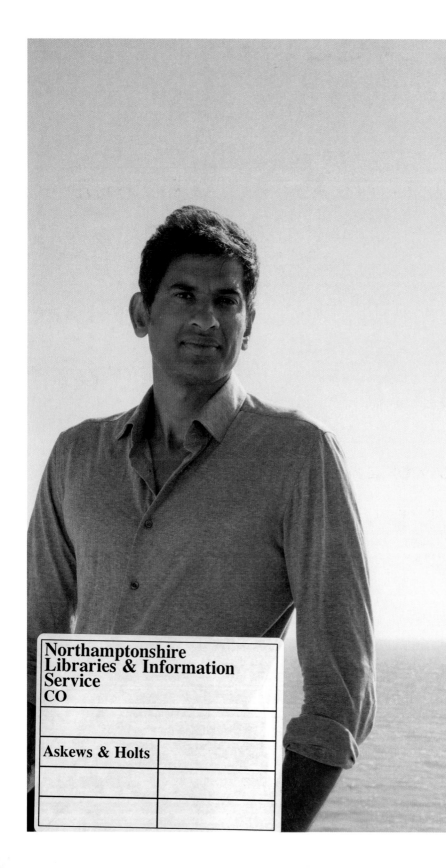

DR RANGAN CHATTERJEE

THE FOUR PILLAR PLAN

How to Relax, Eat, Move and Sleep Your Way to a Longer, Healthier Life

PHOTOGRAPHY BY SUSAN BELL

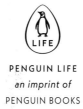

PENGUIN LIFE
an imprint of
PENGUIN BOOKS

PENGUIN LIFE

UK | USA | Canada | Ireland | Australia

India | New Zealand | South Africa

Penguin Life is part of the Penguin Random House group of companies whose addresses can be found at global.penguinrandomhouse.com.

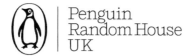

First published 2018
001

Set in Neue Kabel
Colour reproduction by ALTA Image
Printed in Europe by APPL

A CIP catalogue record for this book is available from the British Library

ISBN: 978–0–241–30355–9

www.greenpenguin.co.uk

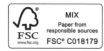

MIX
Paper from
responsible sources
FSC® C018179

Penguin Random House is committed to a sustainable future for our business, our readers and our planet. This book is made from Forest Stewardship Council® certified paper.

For my Dad, you have influenced me
in more ways than you ever knew.
I wish you were still here.

CONTENTS

Introduction   8

How to Use This Book   14

RELAX   16

1. Me-time every day   22

2. The screen-free Sabbath   36

3. Keep a gratitude journal   44

4. Practise stillness daily   47

5. Reclaim your dining table   66

EAT   72

1. De-normalize sugar
   (and retrain your taste buds)   80

2. A new definition of 'five a day'   90

3. Introduce daily micro-fasts   108

4. Drink more water   119

5. Unprocess your diet   124

MOVE   146

1. Walk more   156

2. Become stronger   160

3. Begin regular high-intensity
   interval training   170

4. Movement snacking   178

5. Wake up your sleepy glutes   182

SLEEP   200

1. Create an environment of absolute
   darkness   213

2. Embrace morning light   222

3. Create a bedtime routine   232

4. Manage your commotion   238

5. Enjoy your caffeine before noon   244

FINDING YOUR BALANCE   251

Sources and Further Reading   254

Acknowledgements   260

Index   262

Notes   268

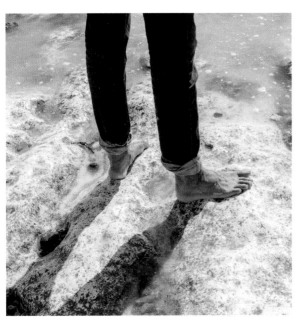

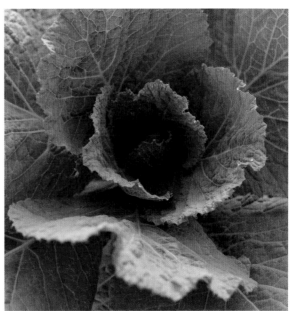

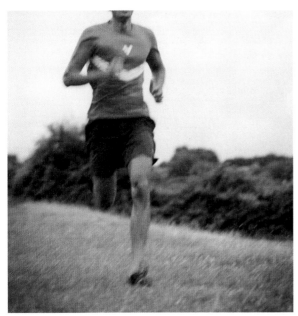

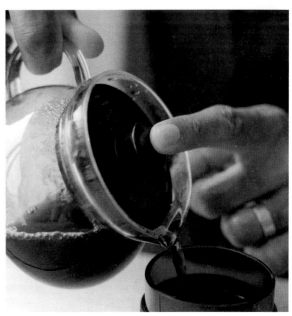

INTRODUCTION

We are very used to the idea that certain lifestyles are bad for us. We know we shouldn't smoke; we're aware that sitting at a desk for eight hours per day isn't a great idea, and that we should avoid eating lots of sugar. Perhaps a less familiar idea is that our lifestyles can actually be medicine. It's not just that we should avoid bad habits – it's that the right lifestyle and nutrition can actually improve our well-being, reverse our health problems and even make chronic diseases like type 2 diabetes, obesity and depression disappear.

It took a while for this to come into focus for me. A few years into my job as a GP, I realized that I was probably helping only around one-fifth of the patients walking through my door. I could certainly give them a drug to suppress their symptoms, but I was failing to get to the actual root cause of their problems. The trouble with the way we both think about health and practise medicine is this: we forget that the human body is one big connected system. If a patient presents to us with symptoms of depression, the usual textbook diagnosis is that it's a psychological condition, caused by a chemical imbalance in the brain. That will almost certainly lead to the prescription of an antidepressant. What I found was that depression, along with many other conditions, could just as easily be driven by poor diet, high stress levels, a lack of physical activity or, even more likely, a combination of all three. Similarly with eczema: the textbook tells us to prescribe a steroid cream for the rash, but the rash is just a symptom. There's little awareness that the causes of eczema are many, among them an overreactive

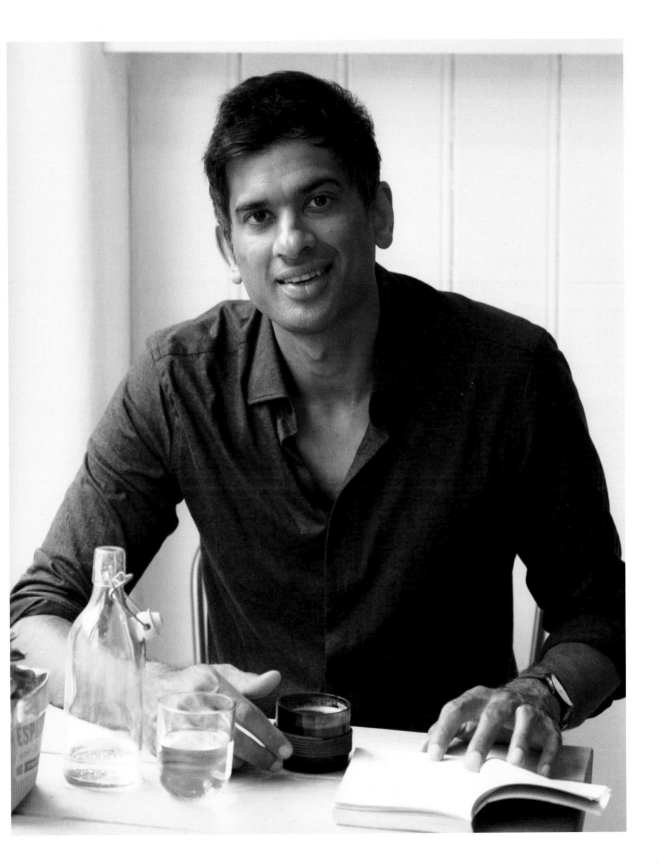

This is why I believe that the future of medicine will be about more doctors being super-generalists, rather than super-specialists. Just as our understanding of the human body is evolving, so the practice of medicine will also need to evolve.

immune system which in turn may be caused by food intolerance, abnormal gut bacteria or even high stress levels. Why not treat these problems, rather than the rash, and get rid of the eczema for good?

The fact is, the body doesn't work as the simplistic and reductionist textbook expects it to. It's a highly evolved biological mechanism that is completely interconnected. This is why I was only managing to treat around 20 per cent of my patients. All too often, a symptom in one domain might actually have a cause in an area of the body that our medical training just doesn't tell us to look at. This is why I believe that the future of medicine will be about more doctors being super-generalists, rather than super-specialists. Just as our understanding of the human body is evolving, so the practice of medicine will also need to evolve. Good health occurs outside the doctor's surgery – not inside. Our lifestyles themselves are often the best medicine.

I'll give you an example of how the current way we view health is tripping us up – with potentially very serious consequences. For years, doctors have struggled to treat a condition called chronic fatigue syndrome. This has led to it being one of the most frustrating conditions that we see, because we don't seem to be able to help. I think the reason medical researchers are struggling so badly to find an effective treatment is that they're reseeking a single cause and a single cure. But my research into the interconnectedness of the body has convinced me there *is* no single cause of this condition. I believe that patients who develop chronic fatigue syndrome are usually experiencing multiple problems, and in order to help them we need to address them all.

Our bodies, and the minds that interact with them, are systems of almost unparalleled complexity. I'm heartened to see some research on this basis is now being conducted into 'incurable' conditions such as Alzheimer's. It's early days yet, and a lot more work needs to be done, but in that area at least it's beginning to look as if the multipronged approach I endorse could achieve promising outcomes. I call such an approach 'progressive medicine'. It's the idea that we need to look at as many factors as possible when examining what creates wellness or illness. Because the body is so connected, with relatively distant parts of it affecting each other, the cause (or causes) of any particular illness might not be immediately obvious.

That this 'interconnected' view of health is presenting good outcomes comes as no surprise to me. Back in my surgery in Manchester, it has produced some truly eye-opening results. By taking this view, I find myself prescribing medications that merely address symptoms far less frequently than I used to. Today, I'm much more likely to prescribe a diet high in healthy fats, some meditation and more physical activity than a mood-altering drug for depression. In prescribing small lifestyle adjustments that promote rest and relaxation, encourage better sleep and diet and get people moving, I have managed to reverse type 2 diabetes, get rid of depression, eliminate irritable bowel syndrome, lower blood pressure, reduce menopausal symptoms without the use of hormones, conquer insomnia, help people lose weight, get rid of severe migraines and even reverse autoimmune conditions – all without the use of any medication. We're all familiar with the idea that lifestyle can be the cause of disease. What's not common knowledge is that a change in lifestyle can also be the treatment and prevent us from getting sick in the first place.

The basic idea is simple. Because every of part our body affects, to a greater or lesser degree, pretty much every other part, we need to take a much more rounded view of treatment, one that considers every aspect of the patient's daily life. How well do they sleep? What do they eat? Are they sedentary at work? Are they constantly consulting their smartphone or tablet? This is what I call the 'threshold effect'. The connected system that is in the human body can deal with multiple insults in various places – up to a point. And then the system begins to break down. The point at which it breaks down is our own unique personal threshold. When talking to patients, I liken it to juggling. Most of us can juggle two balls, even three or four. But when we throw that fifth one in, *all* the balls get dropped. We get sick. That sickness might manifest itself as a skin complaint or a blood-sugar problem or a mood disorder or difficulty sleeping. These complaints are signals that things – usually more than one – are going wrong elsewhere in the body. My approach prioritizes the cause over the symptoms.

The point of this book is to give you a simple, actionable plan to do the same. I want to go beyond the sort of health advice we've all been reading about for so long – beyond the fad diets and the quick-fix exercise programmes. We have overcomplicated health – I want to simplify it.

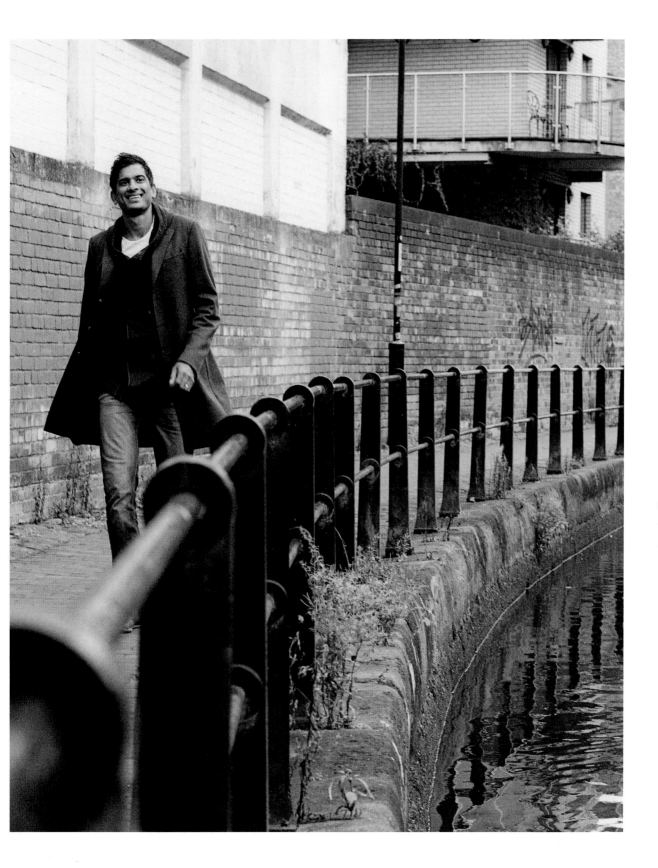

HOW TO USE THIS BOOK

There are four main elements, or pillars, to *The Four Pillar Plan*. The aim of the book is to examine and improve the manner in which you Relax, Eat, Move and Sleep. For each pillar I have set out five ways you might do this, summarized in the table below. The idea is to create balance across *all* the pillars – it is *not* about perfection in each individual one.

I would much rather you score 2 in every pillar, giving you a total score of 8, rather than 5 out of 5 in two separate pillars, giving you a higher score of 10. The numerical score might be smaller but the balance would be greater, and this is the real point of the book.

RELAX

1. Me-time every day

2. Weekly screen-free Sabbath

3. Keep a gratitude journal

4. A daily practice of stillness

5. Eat one meal per day around a table – without an e-device

EAT

1. De-normalize sugar (and retrain your taste buds)

2. Eat five different vegetables every day

3. Eat all your food within a twelve-hour window

4. Drink eight glasses of water per day

5. Unprocess your diet by avoiding any food product that contains more than five ingredients

Achieving balance is what will lead to the biggest improvements and, most importantly, the sustainable ones. This is designed to be a whole-life plan rather than a quick-fix gimmick.

For most of my patients, most of the time, scoring 3 in each pillar resulting in a total score of 12, seems to be about right. It is simply impossible, however, for me to say what will be the right amount for you. Some of you will need to do more, some can get away with less.

It is also possible to take each pillar in isolation. You may feel, for example, that your diet and exercise are already dialled in, whereas your sleep needs more attention. If so, feel free to go straight to that individual pillar and start there. You do not have to go through the book in sequential order. I would prefer you to personalize it to suit your own life.

Give equal priority to every pillar, and proceed at a pace that is comfortable for you.

MOVE

1. Walk at least 10,000 steps per day

2. Do a form of strength training twice a week

3. Do a form of high-intensity interval training twice a week

4. Make a habit of exercise snacking

5. Do daily glute exercises to help wake them up

SLEEP

1. Create an environment of absolute darkness

2. Spend at least twenty minutes outside every morning

3. Create a bedtime routine

4. Manage your commotion

5. Enjoy your caffeine before noon

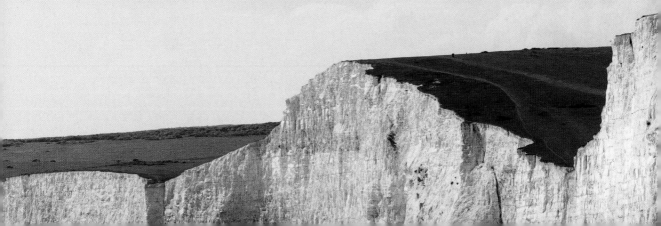

What I'm about to say probably sounds far-fetched, but here it is. The health problems of the majority of patients I see – yes, the *majority* – are driven entirely by their lifestyle. It's not cuts or bruises or bacteria or a fungus or a virus or some tumour or hereditary disorder that's the source of their pain, but the way they're choosing to live. Their conditions are very often exacerbated by the fact that they're super busy. They wake up fully stressed, rush to get the kids ready, do the school run, come back, try to juggle their jobs and their home life. On top of that, they might have other family members who require care and attention. From the moment they open their eyes, it's all go, go, go. Then, when their kids are finally in bed, they're straight into their emails or social media. At no point in the day are they just chilling out, or even alone. Everything they do is for someone else. When I mention this in surgery, they roll their eyes, telling me, 'But I just don't have time for me.' To which I reply, 'Well that, right there, is your problem.'

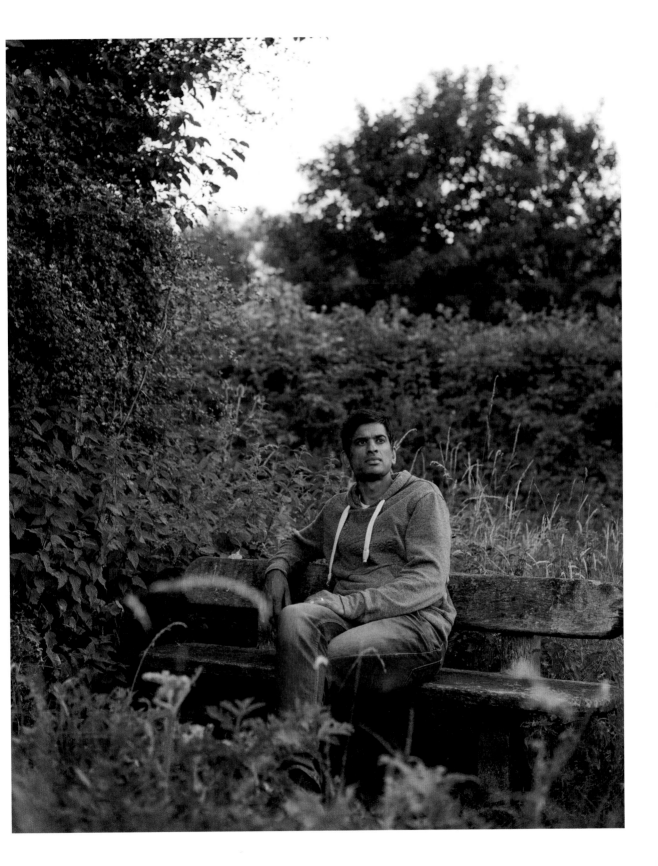

GIVE YOURSELF PERMISSION TO RELAX

I never thought that, as a doctor, I'd have to give anyone permission to do anything. I see my patients as adults who can make their own decisions. But daily experience has taught me that, when it comes to relaxation, a surprising number of people don't get any. So here I am, giving you doctor's orders: I want you to give daily relaxation as high a priority as food, movement and sleep. I think our lack of routine switch-off time is one of the most pressing issues in modern society. For your health, it could hardly be more critical.

In this Relax pillar, as in the other three, you'll find five different interventions. Whilst you are reading through them, start to think about which ones resonate the most, and which ones you might be able to introduce into your life right away. I would love you to adopt at least three, but if that seems too daunting, build up to it by taking on one at a time. I'm the type who's always desperate to jump in and attempt the lot, but we're all different, and it's really important that you find your own pace. It really doesn't matter *how* you get there, as long as you get there.

The Relax pillar is the one I struggle with the most. However, despite many challenges along the way, I've seen the benefits in my own life. I've also seen it in my practice. Potential gains include:

- Weight loss
- Improved resilience
- Reduced feelings of stress
- Improved ability to cope
- More balanced outlook
- Less road rage
- Improved ability to sleep
- More restorative sleep
- Better concentration

There is a reason why I've started this book with the Relax pillar. It's the one that most often gets ignored, both by the public and also by the plethora of quick-fix health books that are out there. Which intervention should you start with? I genuinely don't believe there's much between them but, if you made me choose, the two I would prioritize are the first – carving out some me-time every single day – and the fourth – a daily practice of stillness. The benefits are not only immense but also can be rapid, which will help you engage with the others.

From the moment of her entrance the luncheon party

extravagantly receptive.

Mrs Stitch directed upon him some of her piercing shafts of charm she found him first numb, then dazzled, then have doubled the sum to purchase his release. Thus when gay, to this harrowing experience, he would really, now, qualities that had exposed him in the middle of a busy announced. He was a stranger in these parts; it was up each time the door was opened and sat down at the Megalopolitan Newspaper Corporation would have difficulties to recognize the uneasy figure which time to time and had disregarded him. His subordinates did not know and Lord Copper, had been admitted from Lord Copper, however, who normally launched at one, was waiting with some impatience. Various men and car in a garage half-way to Bethnal Green, and return to (having been obliged by press of traffic to leave her little Curzon Street by means of the Underground railway). ten minutes to two. It was precisely at this time, simul- When Lady Metroland said half past one she meant

'No?'

'Foregoners. Algy's been sacking ten spies a day for weeks. It's a grossly overcrowded profession. Why don't you go as a war correspondent?'

'Could you fix it?'

'I don't see why not. After all, you've been to Pata- gonia. I should think they would jump at you. You're sure you really want to go?'

'Quite sure.'

'Well, I'll see what I can do. I'm meeting Lord Copper at lunch today at Margot's,' I'll try and bring the subject up.'

1. ME-TIME EVERY DAY

Every day, for at least fifteen minutes, be selfish,
and enjoy some time for you.

For at least fifteen minutes, every day, and more if possible, stop everything and be utterly selfish. Stop treating 'relaxation' as something that you do – or, more likely, don't do – when everything else has been dealt with. *Choose* to relax. Make it a triple-underlined part of your schedule. Set an alarm. What will you do? Will you visit a local cafe, buy a coffee and indulge in a trashy magazine? Will you sit in a room with the lights off, listening to your favourite piece of music? Will you enjoy a relaxing bath? It's entirely up to you. But there are three rules. Firstly, it must be something unashamedly for you and you alone. Secondly, it must not be an activity that involves your smartphone, tablet or computer. Thirdly, you're not allowed to feel guilty about it.

CORTISOL SURGE

Had you told me this a few years ago, I wouldn't have believed it, but simply setting aside little moments every day can make a massive difference to your health. There are many reasons why these breaks make a difference, but a principal one is that they can help us to switch off our overactive stress response. Now, we all have cortisol in our bodies, and we all need it. Cortisol is a hormone, and a hormone is a chemical messenger. When we feel hungry, satiated, aroused, angry and so on, it's because particular hormones are surging around our bloodstreams. Cortisol has been identified as one of our principal stress-response hormones. Hormone levels tend to spike and fall at different times of the day, in natural cycles, and also rise and fall in response to the things that are happening to us. Our cortisol level surges when we're stressed.

Contrary to popular belief, stress isn't necessarily bad for us. We've evolved to experience stress for all sorts of good reasons. An onrush of stress primes our minds and bodies to tackle a sudden problem head-on. But we're designed to experience stress in short bursts. When we endure it for a sustained period, it becomes a problem. To find out why this is, we must cast our view back hundreds of thousands of years. Humans are the product of an extremely gradual process of evolution that took place over many millennia. Our bodies and brains have been specialized, not for modern living in towns and cities, but for existence in roaming hunter-gatherer groups of no more than 150 people. Because this kind of evolution occurs so slowly, our ancient systems haven't caught up with twenty-first-century life. Our machinery for responding to and dealing with stress is still largely prehistoric. And that mismatch between the ancient biological technology we have in our bodies and the complex, ultra-modern lives we're living can have some pretty nasty effects.

NORMAL CORTISOL RHYTHM THROUGHOUT THE DAY

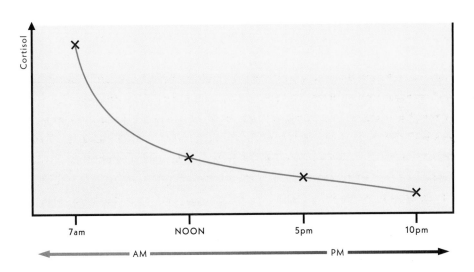

Imagine what kind of stresses our bodies were designed to cope with all those years ago. If we were attacked by a lion, say, that experience would be terrifying but it would also be short lived. Either we'd have run away and escaped, or killed the lion, and the danger would have passed, or we'd have been killed. That's the kind of event our stress equipment has been built to deal with. Our autonomic nervous system is a bodily network around which signals and instructions are transmitted, and there are two parts to it, the sympathetic system and the parasympathetic. Cortisol works by activating our sympathetic nervous system. This is our fight-or-flight response. And what I'm seeing in my practice is that people are *constantly* in fight-or-flight mode. They're spending their days with their cortisol levels continuously ramped right up, their sympathetic nervous systems activated. They're not being attacked by a lion, they're being attacked by their life.

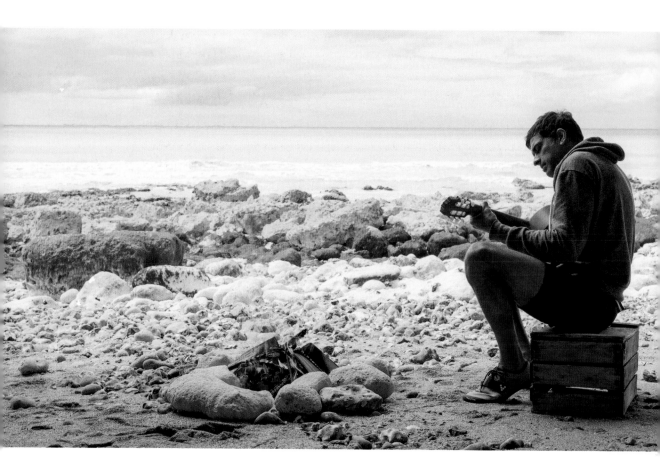

THE TWO PARTS OF THE AUTONOMIC NERVOUS SYSTEM

Our autonomic nervous system regulates our automatic processes – the things we do without consciously thinking like breathing and digestion.

One branch of this system, the sympathetic nervous system, causes the body to release stress-response hormones such as noradrenaline and cortisol. It causes your heart rate to quicken, your lung tubes to widen, your muscles to contract, your pupils to dilate and it switches off digestion. It helps divert energy away from processes in our body such as digestion that are not necessary for our survival. It helps us release energy from our muscles and lowers immune system function. In the short term this helps us deal with the stress, but if activated long term this response can become problematic.

In the modern world, this fight-or-flight system activates when we're rushing to meet a deadline, getting stressed on our commute, leaving late for the school run or putting ourselves through a tough workout. This response can be managed, as long as we take steps to balance it out with rest and relaxation.

This rest and relaxation involves the other branch of our nervous system, which is the parasympathetic. It works at a much slower rate than the sympathetic branch. When it's activated our saliva production increases, digestive enzymes are released, our heart rate drops and our muscles relax. It allows us to digest food appropriately, destress and sleep soundly.

To help manage the stress of modern life we should be encouraging the activation of the parasympathetic nervous system – all five interventions in the Relax pillar will help you do just that.

CORTISOL STEAL

This is harmful for a number of reasons. Firstly, there's something called the 'cortisol steal'. All the hormones in your body are made from the same basic stuff, which is called LDL cholesterol. We naturally have a limited supply of LDL cholesterol and, when things are working well, it all gets portioned off nicely, so there's enough to go round – enough to make your oestrogen, your progesterone, your testosterone – and also your cortisol. But what happens when you're in one of these long-term states of stress is that cortisol steals the other hormones' LDL cholesterol. Because it thinks you're under attack, and in a state of crisis, your body prioritizes the generation of cortisol. It thinks you need it to cope with the drama and just makes more and more of it. That upsets the finely tuned balance of hormones in your body.

This leads to a wide variety of problems. Clinicians know we're currently seeing an increase in numbers of men with low testosterone. This impacts things like sex drive, muscular strength, energy levels and even risk of chronic disease, and testosterone prescriptions now cost the NHS something like £20 million per year. I'm convinced the underlying problem in many of these cases is stress, leading to overproduction of cortisol at the expense of other hormones, of which testosterone is just one.

But it's not just the cortisol steal we need to be concerned about. When we're constantly stressed, our bodies respond as if we're under attack, going into a kind of emergency mode and diverting resources to the processes most necessary for survival. To take just one example, digestion switches off. When you're dealing with a lion flying at your head, the efficient processing of lunch is just an unnecessary diversion. A more pressing need is the generation of instant energy in your bloodstream.

In the short term this is great, but when this becomes long term it creates a problem. It can lead to weight gain and sleep disruption and exhausts the immune system. Remember, all of this is happening because the body thinks it's under attack all day. Whilst there are an infinite number of stressors in our environment, there's only one main stress response. Your body can't tell the difference between emotional stress, physical stress and nutritional stress. It can't tell the difference between the stress of missing a mortgage payment or the stress you feel when someone's been rude to you on Facebook. To your system, it's all just a lion flying at your head and it reacts in the same way in every case.

IMPACT ON YOUR DIGESTIVE SYSTEM

You know when you get that mid-morning hunger surge? You've had your bowl of sugar-coated cereal, your blood sugar's gone up, then mid-morning it's crashed. You're starving. You're shaky. You need something to eat. When your blood sugar falls suddenly like this, that's another stressor, another lion at your head. It can send your cortisol and adrenaline soaring. So even something as simple as choosing the wrong breakfast can tip your body into this emergency state. Then what happens? Not only are you likely to go hunting in your fridge or biscuit tin for some more bad food, your digestion is suppressed, so it's a double hit on the weight gain. This is another example of why it's crucial that we view the body as a massively connected system. One potential cause – in this case, a sugary breakfast – can have multiple effects, including stress, the cortisol steal and weight gain.

IMPACT ON YOUR IMMUNE SYSTEM

But that's not all. When your body thinks it's under attack, it puts your immune system into an emergency state. This makes perfect sense from an evolutionary perspective. Imagine if you managed to survive that lion attack by fighting it off. It's likely you'd be left with cuts that were prone to infection – the animal would've had nasty bugs in its claws or saliva and your wounds pick up dirt from your environment. This is why your immune system needs to go into a peak state. We call this heightened immune response 'inflammation' and, again, we're not supposed to be in this state for an extended period of time. Chronic inflammation (in medical parlance, any nasty condition that hangs around for too long is referred to as 'chronic') underpins pretty much every single degenerative disease that we have, including heart attacks, strokes and even Alzheimer's disease.

A 2016 paper published by researchers at King's College London highlighted just one of the ways inflammation can have a surprising impact on the massively connected body. They showed a remarkable link between inflammation and depression. The scientists suggested we can predict which patients suffering from depression will respond to conventional antidepressants by giving them blood tests that show their levels of inflammation. Crucially, they found that patients with high degrees of inflammation do not respond to conventional antidepressants. The results confirm what other scientific research has been suggesting for years – that depression itself can be a symptom of biological changes in the body that are driven by inflammation. This is why antidepressants don't work for these patients.

If your problem is not in your brain – if it's actually inflammation in your body – what's the point in giving you a drug that's going to tweak something in your head?

Think about how astonishing this is. If someone is depressed, the textbook medicine approach points our clinical gaze at possible struggles they're having in their life, or past traumas, or perhaps even chemical problems in their brain. But the root cause might just as easily be inflammation that's caused by having too much cortisol charging about their system, for too long. This is how healthcare needs to evolve – into an era of progressive medicine characterized by the growing awareness that the name of a disease can often tell us very little about the actual cause. 'Depression' is simply a name we give to a collection of symptoms – the word itself doesn't tell us anything about the root of the problem.

Understanding all this is increasingly transforming the way I practise medicine. Recently I was consulted by Miranda, a fifty-two-year-old whom I hadn't seen for about six months. She had been following all my advice but now had seemed to plateau, and was not improving any further. I spent a long time chatting to her to try to figure out why. As we got into her story, it became clear that she had no time for herself at all. She was always on the go and she never stopped. When I put this to her, she said, 'Family life is just stressful.' I tested her saliva. As I expected, her cortisol levels were through the roof. I kicked myself for not going down this path sooner. Stress is now a critical line of investigation I pursue in relation to a huge array of complaints.

STRESS AND THE MENOPAUSE

I've treated menopausal difficulties in women by helping them deal more effectively with their stress levels. These women have a problem with their hormones, namely oestrogen and progesterone. The textbook medicine approach often results in doctors prescribing a course of hormone replacement therapy (HRT), which can comprise various combinations of these female hormones. Not only is HRT a cost burden on the NHS, it can also have some unpleasant side-effects, including bloating, swelling, nausea, cramps and even vaginal bleeding. There are also ongoing concerns about possible increased risks of ovarian cancer, breast cancer and blood clots.

There's no doubt that HRT often works, but is it always necessary? If the patient is stressed, most of her body's LDL cholesterol is likely going straight into making cortisol. This means there's less of it left to make oestrogen and progesterone. HRT deals with the symptom, but why not go to the root cause instead? Normalizing cortisol levels – whether through meditation (see page 47) or from sectioning off some daily me-time, or even from switching to a wholefood diet (which helps reduce the nutritional stress caused by low-quality foods) – very often alleviates menopausal symptoms entirely.

STRESS AND THE GUT

I once treated a forty-year-old woman who had a bad case of Crohn's disease using these principles. Crohn's is a nasty bowel complaint and she'd been getting painful stomach cramps and kept needing to go to the toilet. Nothing seemed to be helping her and she'd reached the point where she was losing patience with her specialist. Eventually, she came in to see me. I made some changes to her diet that helped for a while, but she quickly plateaued. I couldn't understand why this was, so I decided to delve deeper. I soon realized she literally had nothing in her daily life for herself. Everything was to do with her kids and her husband. She was going at full speed all the time, never putting herself first. 'Are there any other medications I should be trying?' she asked. 'What else should I do with my diet?'

'You know what?' I said. 'I'm going to try something completely different. I'm going to give you another appointment in a month. In the meantime, here's what I want you to do.' I took out my notepad and wrote a list of three things. 'Two fifteen-minute periods for you per day. A walk every morning. And find something to do, at least twice a week, that you love and that you do just for you.'

After falling out with her specialist, this was the last thing she wanted to hear. I could see it written all over her face – she thought I was reverting to soft, woolly, paternalistic medicine. Perhaps she even felt patronized. She had a serious illness and she expected serious medicine. 'And what about supplements?' she asked me crossly. 'What about medication?'

'That's it,' I said. 'That's all I want you to do.' I pushed the note towards her. 'This is your prescription.'

Now, I knew this patient very well. Despite her suspicions, she trusted me and I was hopeful that she'd at least give it a chance. When she came back four weeks later, I was delighted. She told me she'd joined a salsa class, which was something she'd been thinking about for years but had never done because she didn't think she had time. She'd also started going out for a walk in the mornings. She'd spent time in her living room, leaving her phone and laptop on the kitchen counter, just sitting and listening to music for fifteen minutes. We completed a medical symptom questionnaire, which is designed to measure objectively the effects of illness with questions such as how often she had stomach cramps or bowel movements. Even I was astonished to find her Crohn's symptoms had reduced by 50 per cent. This kind of reduction in a four-week time frame, for a condition as complex and serious as Crohn's, is simply incredible.

What, to the outside observer, might be even more surprising is that the symptoms of Crohn's are located in the gut and none of the interventions I gave her seemed to have anything to do with that part of her body. But I know that if cortisol is up, it won't just affect how calm you're feeling, it will affect your gut function. Not only that but your inflammation markers go up, and the way your cytokines, which are chemicals that send messages within the immune system, behave changes. What does all this tell us? It tells us that the body is massively connected. Although she had a gut problem, her non-switching-off problem was making it worse. Of course, I'm not saying this will work for every Crohn's patient. There's simply no trial that says that this is *the* way to treat it – and nor is there likely to be. But that's not because interventions like this don't work. It's because everyone who has Crohn's is different.

I feel strongly that, as a doctor, I should try to follow my own advice and, by and large, I do. One of my patients, a firefighter, once told me the only reason he was going to do as I suggested was that I was the first doctor he'd seen who actually practised what he preached.

CYTOKINES

Cytokines are proteins released by the immune system. They work as messengers, taking the information being put out by the immune system around the body. They are essential to immune system function and are involved with coordinating the initiation, maintenance and resolution of all immune responses. Maintaining a delicate balance in the level of these communicators is vital for health.

The immune system releases cytokines in response not only to infections and traumatic accidents but also to triggers such as stress, food and exercise.

Their release is tightly regulated as their impact can be severe: some of them cause inflammation while others have the opposite effect. Some, including interleukin 6, can serve both functions in different situations.

I'll be honest, though – in the past, I have struggled to find time for me. But not any more: I have built me-time into my daily routine. At my last practice, midway through morning surgery I allowed time for a fifteen-minute walk. Reception knew not to book anyone in between 10.15 and 10.30. Even if there were patients waiting I would still stop everything and go for a stroll. At first my manager wasn't at all happy – 'Why is he doing this when he ought to be seeing patients?' – but she quickly realized that I would still see as many patients as anyone else, if not more.

Recently, I have re-engaged with cooking whilst having a favourite CD on – it is amazing how relaxing this can be. What can you do to give you your daily dose?

I prioritize me-time. It's scheduled into my daily timetable. In today's world there's *always* something else to do – an email to send, a Facebook feed to scroll, a tweet to reply to. It's never-ending. That's why you need to make a proactive decision to prioritize it.

One of my recent patients, forty-four-year-old Suzanne, was busy juggling mother-hood and a part-time job. When she told me she didn't have time for herself, I said to her, 'Suzanne, after you've dropped the kids off, you go straight to the shops, back home, straight to emails and then you're go-go-go all day until it is time to pick them up. What would happen if your car broke down? You'd stop for an hour or so whilst you waited for the breakdown service. That would enforce your switch-off time. You'd still get everything done afterwards, wouldn't you?' This resonated with her. She made it a rule every day after the kids were dropped off to go for a phone-free fifteen-minute walk, rain or shine. Six weeks later, she felt like a different person. She was less stressed throughout the day, and, counter-intuitively, actually became *more* productive and got more things done. This tiny change had a huge impact.

Just by making space for yourself for fifteen minutes per day, as Suzanne did, you can help normalize your cortisol levels. Your body will be reminded what it's like not to feel under attack. I contend that modern living, even if it's something as simple and common as your email inbox overflowing, is stressful. *I* find it stressful. And what's the downside, in our busy culture, of actually trying this? There's none whatsoever. Ironically it's the people who say they don't have time for these interventions who need to do them the most.

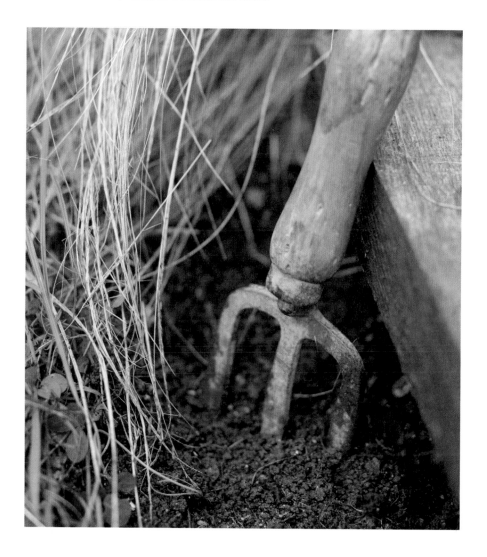

EXAMPLES OF PHONE-FREE ME-TIME
YOU MIGHT CONSIDER:

Having a bath ✓	Playing music ✓
Going for a walk ✓	Gardening ✓
Sitting in a cafe having a drink ✓	Cooking with your favourite album playing, or in silence ✓
Sitting on a park bench relaxing ✓	Painting ✓
Reading a magazine ✓	Dancing ✓
Reading a book ✓	Fifteen minutes of yoga or Tai Chi ✓
Singing ✓	Relaxing at home, with or without music ✓

You can also bring in components of your daily stillness practice (see page 47).

2. THE SCREEN-FREE SABBATH

Every Sunday, turn off your screens and live your day offline.

It was a typically hectic day at my Oldham practice, at the end of a Monday afternoon, and I was running late. In the NHS, we're allotted ten minutes for each patient and it's easy to find your appointments running into each other. Your only hope for getting back on track is to luck into seeing a few people you can deal with speedily. This is what I was hoping would happen last summer when a sixteen-year-old named Devon came in, accompanied by his mum. But the moment they sat down, I realized this would be anything but a quick one. 'Dr Chatterjee,' said the mother, struggling slightly to get the words out. 'On Saturday night, Devon cut his wrists with a knife.'

'On purpose?' I asked.

'On purpose,' she nodded. 'I had to take him to A&E. The psychiatrist there said we should see you for antidepressants. We're here for the prescription.'

It would've taken thirty seconds to write them a note for Prozac and send them on their way. But something stopped me. We started chatting and slowly Devon began to open up. I knew I had patients who were being delayed, but I also knew I couldn't do this boy a disservice. I needed to understand, why would a sixteen-year-old boy, from a seemingly well-balanced family, start self-harming out of nowhere?

As I probed, I discovered that he felt like a misfit at school, partly because of his hobbies and partly because of his appearance. I started asking him about social media usage.

'Do you go on it quite a lot?'

'I go on it loads,' he grinned.

'Do you use it in bed at night?'

'Yeah, I'll go on Facebook, I'll be texting.'

'Look,' I said, 'I'm wondering whether your use of social media is contributing to this in a small way.' His face fell and his mother looked dubious. 'Would you consider reducing it?'

'Why?' he said.

'I'm not sure it's helping your mental health. Your self-harming is a symptom. I want to find out what's causing it. An hour before bed, how about if you just switch your phone off? Do you think you could do that?'

'Errm,' he said.

'I'll tell you what. Why don't you give it a go for a week? If you're still feeling the same, I'll write you that script.'

I imagine that some of you may have been getting palpitations just from reading the title of this chapter. I know how you feel. I used to feel that way too. It's not that I'm against social media or the internet – not all. But I am seeing a huge rise in problems that stem from their use. This is hardly surprising, given their rapid ascent and infiltration into every aspect of our lives. It's now thought that there are more mobile devices on the planet than people – truly remarkable. Some of us – me included – can find it hard to leave our e-devices alone for more than ten minutes. If I'm playing with my kids on a Sunday and my phone's nearby, there's a constant nagging impulse to look at it. And I know for a fact that I am not the only one. We're encouraged to keep on checking our feeds, to see how many likes or followers we have, or to update ourselves on the latest gossip. We have even started looking at our work emails on our days off. This contributes to the wider problem, one that's become exponentially more problematic since the introduction of smartphones. We are all finding it harder to switch off. When we open our eyes in the morning, instead of letting our bodies gradually awaken we're straight onto Twitter or Facebook or Snapchat, or whatever the latest social platform is, letting this constant stream of noise into our brains. And this noise is a huge problem. Five years ago, I was convinced that the root cause of most of the complaints I saw in my practice was poor diet. Now I'm convinced it's stress.

SMARTPHONE ADDICTION

There's quite a bit of controversy out there about whether or not we can, in a truly clinical sense, say that the use of smartphones can be addictive. But real-world experience has left me in little doubt. One 2014 study of 2,000 people painted a disturbing portrait of the average user. We check our phones 221 times a day, starting at around 7:31 a.m., when we'll look at Facebook, read the news and check the weather before we've even got out of bed. By the time we go to sleep, we'll have spent three hours and sixteen minutes on our device. An even more alarming statistic from the US estimates that the average user touches their phone 2,617 times per day.

A large part of why these numbers are so ridiculously high is the fact that we're now constantly contactable, and subject to a ceaseless barrage of emails, calls and texts. But what's also happened, in the last ten or so years, is the beginning of an unhealthy 'selfie' culture that feeds our phone addiction even more. Studies suggest that humans spend as much as 40 per cent of our speech time informing others about our own subjective experiences. It's believed that doing this fires up neural pathways associated with reward and activates addiction centres in the brain such as the nucleus accumbens. It's easy to see how a few selfies with mindless updates on Facebook, Instagram and Snapchat can start to create a feedback loop in your brain where you crave more and more of the same. My experience has been that, just like many drugs, the more you use your smartphone, the more addicted you become.

Studies suggest that humans spend as much as 40 per cent of our speech time informing others about our own subjective experiences. It's believed that doing this fires up neural pathways associated with reward and activates addiction centres in the brain such as the nucleus accumbens.

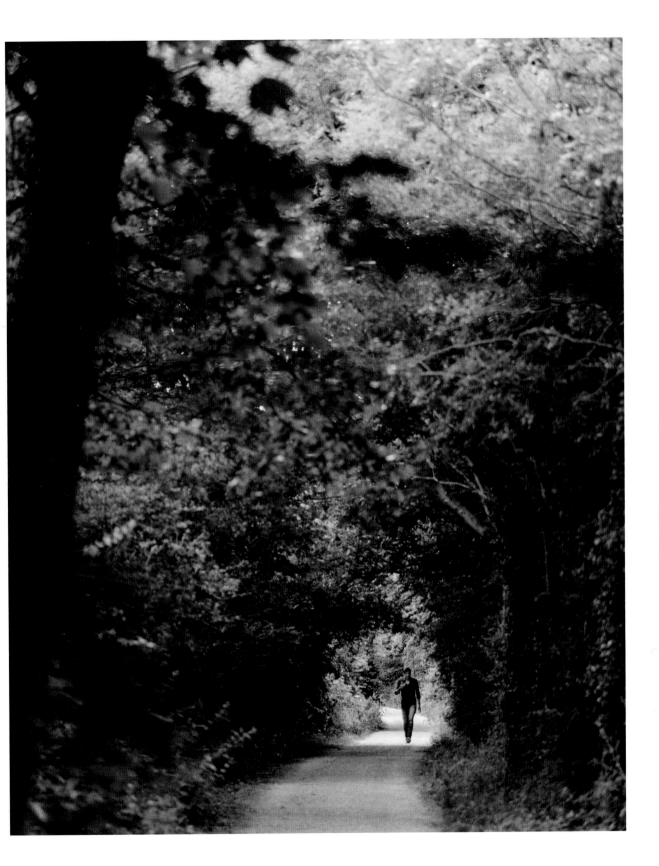

We've evolved to enjoy social validation. We're highly social creatures. Just as the company making Mars bars takes advantage of the fact we've evolved to love sweetness, so social media takes advantage of the fact we've evolved to crave the approval of others. But, just like the 7.7 teaspoons of sugar you'll find in a Mars bar, we were never designed to have so much of it. When the massively connected human machine was evolving, we expected to have sugar now and again, especially in the summer. This is what that machine still expects. It's what it was designed for. We also used to have the tribe applauding us once every now and then when we did something truly selfless or brave. But we now live in an age when we can have all these things all the time. We're overusing all our inbuilt evolutionary mechanisms. And you'd have to be naive to think there aren't going to be consequences.

An additional problem is what psychologists who study social media are now describing as 'perfectionist presentation'. People don't tend to post on the bad parts of their day, they tend to focus on the good stuff. This creates a false reality in which it can seem like everyone else is much more successful, and enjoying a much better life, than we are. We all tend to compare our lives to other people's and judge ourselves accordingly. These are automatic processes. We can't help it. In vulnerable adolescents, this can be an easy road to stress and depression. It can be just as harmful in adults.

RESET YOUR RELATIONSHIP

One way in which you can start to reset your relationship with electronic media is by altering how you use your smartphone. I have tried this over the past eighteen months and immediately felt the benefits. Taking notifications off your phone is a great place to start. All your apps are still there and functioning, but every time someone likes an Instagram comment you've liked, or checks your profile on Linkedin, you don't get a notification. You could extend this further by turning off the auto-sync on your email inbox. Now you have to physically request your email inbox to refresh.

I used to be addicted to the sight of a new notification on the screen of my phone. Now I don't see them. I can pick my phone up to make a call, blissfully unaware that

I have ten new emails waiting for me. This may not sound like much in isolation, but when you think about how many times we look at our phones every day, this adds up to a lot of time. You could even try introducing a 'device box' at home into which everyone in your household has to drop their phone before meals. The possibilities are endless and it is simply impossible for me to say what will end up working for you in the context of your own life. What helps pretty much everyone, however, is making some kind of change, no matter how small. Remember, every time you hear a notification or the ping of a new email you activate reward signals in your brain that leave you craving more.

What I hear again and again from my patients is that they had no idea how great an impact their e-device was having on their lives. There's no down time when you have a smartphone in your pocket. How often do you go for dinner and you're with your partner or best friend, but you're really not with them? How many times have you felt a 'phantom phone buzz' in your trouser pocket? What's *that* about?

Taking regular breaks from his smartphone was quite a novel and scary idea for Devon, but he did it. And when I saw him the following week he told me he felt different. A fortnight later he reported he was sleeping better. We started to reduce his use even further, so he waited for one hour after waking to begin and stopped two hours before bedtime. After about six weeks, I asked him to begin changing his diet, replacing simple sugars such as biscuits, cakes and sugary cereals with healthy, natural fats such as eggs, avocados and nuts (which are needed for hormone production). At the next consultation, he smiled and told me his mood and emotions were much more stable and he was getting anxious less and less often. Six months later I received a letter from his mum, saying that Devon was like a different boy, with friends at school and no more problems, and that I had changed his life. I never did write him that prescription for Prozac.

Can I say that reducing smartphone use alone was what made Devon better? No, I can't. This wasn't an academic study and these weren't laboratory conditions. But I would go as far as saying that reducing his exposure at specific times of the day, combined with the dietary changes, turned his life around. This was a young man whose problems very easily could have been given a label – depression – and treated with medication. And that is happening over and over again in surgeries up and down the country.

CAN YOU GO WITHOUT?

The goal of this intervention is for you to examine, change, and then reset your relationship with your electronic devices. Clearly, it is not my place to tell you how to consume your digital media. That is up to you. My hope is for you to question your current usage; how much of it is what you have chosen and how much of it chose you. Just because smartphones have the functionality of emails, does that mean you have to use it? What happens if you don't?

Many of you, I am sure, will be a little fearful of missing out on something important by not constantly checking your emails. But as a friend of mine recently realized, if your email says you are unavailable, you are unavailable. He realized that by turning them off when he was away, he was controlling his time and stress levels far better, raher than being controlled by his device and by emails from other people (i.e other people's agendas). It's really about trying to use your devices in a way that helps you rather than enslaves you.

For me, one of the hallmarks of the addict is denial. They'll tell themselves, 'Of course I could give up if I really wanted to, I'm completely in control.' But then, when it comes to the crunch, there's always some convenient excuse – 'Oh I would, but I can't today, because blah.' So if you find yourself thinking that smartphone dependency is not a problem in your life, why not try doing without it? See if you can manage it, just for one day per week. Will you find an excuse?

> I created a 7-day digital detox to help you work up to your Screen-Free Sabbath. The goal is to wind down gradually so that, by the time Sunday comes, you will be ready to take the plunge and have an entirely screen-free day. If an entire day is too daunting, start off with half a day – you will still experience positive benefits. If your mobile phone is your only means of communication, why not try having one day per week where you switch off its mobile data and wi-fi connectivity. You will still be contactable by text and phone, yet there will be less temptation to mindlessly surf the internet.

SEVEN-DAY DIGITAL DETOX

MONDAY:
Switch off push notifications on your phone, tablet and laptop

TUESDAY:
Unsubscribe from redundant email lists

WEDNESDAY:
Set your email apps to refresh manually; take emails (or at least work emails) off your phone

THURSDAY:
Device box for meal times – they *must* go in before you sit down

FRIDAY:
Can you switch off your all your e-devices ninety minutes before bed?
Consider disabling your smartphone email inbox until Monday morning

SATURDAY:
Have two one-hour periods during the day where you are e-device free;
see if you can enjoy some special moments without posting them on social media

SUNDAY:
SCREEN-FREE DAY
Live your entire day offline and without screens

3. KEEP A GRATITUDE JOURNAL

Every night, before you go to sleep, write a list of all the things that have gone well for you that day, and all the things you're grateful for.

I discovered this simple but amazingly effective intervention from Charles Poliquin, a brilliant strength coach who's trained Olympic medallists in over twenty different sports. Back when I was a junior doctor I'd read his blogs and think about how useful some of the content would be for many of my patients. I wondered why we hadn't been taught any of these ideas in medical school. I was thrilled to meet him not long ago, and to learn that he has three questions he always asks his daughter before bed. What have you done today to make someone else happy? What has somebody else done today to make you happy? What have you learned? Now the Chatterjee family do it too, except we do it around the dinner table. Even Mum and Dad have to take part. Once you've done it, it's really hard not to feel good. If you've had a bad day, it redirects your thoughts. We have a human tendency to focus on the negatives but the questions challenge us to think, 'Yeah it *was* pretty good, actually,' or, 'I learned XYZ today.' And, more often than not, we leave the dinner table glowing.

What follows is a simplified version of this. Keep a pad and pen by the bed and just spend some time, before you go to sleep, listing all the things that have gone well for you that day, and all the things you're grateful for. I've found this to be really effective at redirecting your thought patterns in the crucial minutes before going to sleep, so that the weight of the world shifts somewhat.

This may sound rather touchy-feely, but it's actually based on sound science. The esteemed US psychologist Martin Seligman, who is one of the founders of happiness studies, or 'positive psychology', had tested a version of this that he calls the 'three blessings' exercise. It involves spending ten minutes before bed writing down three things that went well, no matter how large or small, and also – in order to force you to further 'reflect on and immerse yourself in the good event' – the reason why that thing went well. For Seligman, the act of writing it down is crucial. In a series of well-designed studies, he found that people who do this for a week see rises in their feelings of life satisfaction and a lowering of depression levels. According to Seligman, if you start making this a regular practice, you'll be 'less depressed, happier, and addicted to this exercise six months from now'.

Another US study, led by Chad Burton of Southern Methodist University, had people writing about a positive experience for twenty minutes on three consecutive days. When they were tested three months later, the researchers found the participants enjoyed enhanced mood, less illness and made fewer visits to their doctor. Remember, this was a full quarter of a year after their three days of journaling – a truly remarkable result. And researchers from the University of Manchester found that people who had more feelings of gratitude not only slept better but also had more energy and increased focus.

Of course, religious people have been wise to this clever hack for many centuries. Christians are taught to pray at the end of the day and give thanks. Much of what makes up religious laws are the learned life-lessons in how to live well or maintain some sort of order within populations of people. In the pre-refrigeration age, it would have made sense not to eat pork if you lived in a hot country. These excellent rules for better living became codified as commandments from God. Whilst I'm a Hindu by birth, I'm not pro- or anti- any particular religion. I fully accept and embrace the fact that tied up in each of them is a huge amount of common sense that has been passed from generation to generation. It seems to me that Christians probably found a dose of gratitude at the end of every day increased the quality of their sleep and their state of mind, and that this had plenty of genuinely positive effects on their health and mental well-being. It's only now, in the twenty-first century, that the modern scientific research is proving they were right.

A simple tip is to buy a really nice journal or diary and keep it by your bed. Own it. Love it. Treasure it. For some of my patients, simply buying a little book that they love the look of helps them engage in the process. Whatever you write in it, the important thing is to note down three things every day that you're grateful for. It doesn't need to be complicated. Instead of focusing on the colleague who ignored you in the morning, why not focus on the one who brought you a coffee? Instead of focusing on the hard week you have had, why not think about the fact that it's now the weekend? It could be the three questions that I learned from Charles Poliquin or it can be as simple as the fact you enjoyed your evening meal or you're happy to have a roof over your head. Writing these thoughts down helps subtly shift your focus. And in our modern world where we are bombarded with images of perfection, it is easy for our thoughts to spiral quickly into negativity.

Three things to be grateful for today:

1. ---

----

2. ---

----

3. ---

----

4. PRACTISE STILLNESS DAILY

Make time to practise stillness for at least five minutes daily.

I've been a father for over seven years and it's only been in the last few months that my kids have started sleeping through the night. For such a long time I struggled to cope with the exhaustion that comes with parenting. My energy levels suffered, I'd find it hard to be as attentive as I ought to have been and, sometimes, I'd find myself snapping at those closest to me.

A few years ago, when my son was about three, I tried something new. I'd come downstairs at 5.30 a.m. and meditate for ten minutes. Sometimes I felt, 'What was the point of that?' All I was doing was going through my to-do list for the upcoming day in my head. But on other days, I hit the zone a little more. Slowly, I found my energy levels getting better. I wasn't as reactive – I wasn't responding to things in the instant. I didn't get so cross in the car. My sleep improved. I was able to focus more on my work. Even though, during some sessions, I couldn't switch my mind off at all and was sure the meditation had been a complete waste of time, it didn't seem to matter. The effect remained.

MEDITATION

Meditation is an umbrella term that can cover many things. There are purists who think it has to be done in a traditional way, sitting cross-legged and chanting a mantra, but I think there are many routes leading to the same result. I asked one patient who insisted she couldn't meditate to spend ten minutes every day listening to her favourite song with her eyes closed without any distractions.

'I want you to hear the drum beat, I want you to hear the vocal, I want you to turn the lights off and just be present,' I told her. That, for me, is a musical meditation. Or is it musical 'mindfulness' – a term we've been hearing a lot over the last few years? Well, maybe. Although meditation and mindfulness are not quite the same things, there's a huge amount of overlap. My definition of mindfulness is being attentive and present to what you're doing in the moment. For our purposes, though, I'd like to both broaden these terms and simplify them. Really, it's about stillness.

Looking at it once again in evolutionary terms, when we were hunter-gatherers we would've been used to long periods of boredom or mental stillness – walking to the hunt, waiting for the fire to be hot enough, sitting around at night when there was nothing productive that could be done. Our daily lives would probably

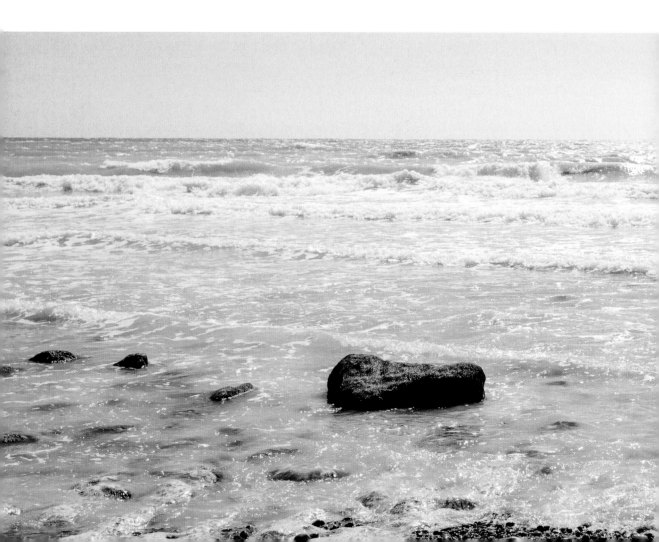

have consisted of lengthy episodes of calmness punctuated by peak moments of stress. This is what our brains and bodies have evolved to expect, but the modern environment just doesn't allow for it. We spend most of our time simply overwhelmed by calls for our attention. This is just one of the ways in which our ordinary daily lives have become poisoned.

And, of course, there are numerous costs. The grey matter in our brains increases when we have regular periods of mindfulness, whilst meditation stimulates neuronal activity, aids sleep quality, aids concentration and lowers blood pressure. More and more research is suggesting that stress can change the composition of the bugs that live in our gut, as well as their relationship with each other. We call these bugs, and all the genetic material contained within them, our 'microbiome'. We're going to be

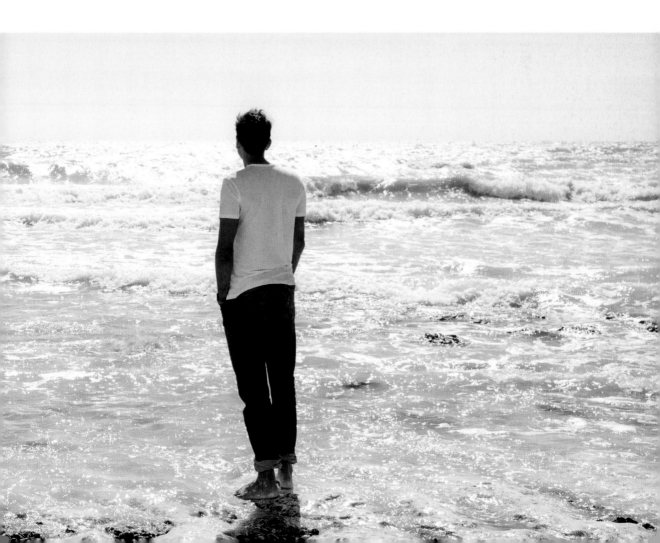

diving deep into the incredible and powerful realm of the microbiome in the Eat pillar, but these trillions of bacteria interact with each other, and with us, and have huge impacts on our health. Their make-up and diversity influence everything from our gut function to our mood. Research on mice suggests that stress changes their microbiome. Whilst we're not mice, it is very reasonable to think that this would be the case in humans too. In this way alone, lowering our stress by practising stillness can have far-reaching effects on the rest of our wellness.

These are the kinds of natural benefits we should be getting automatically, but that we've lost. We're born to thrive. We're born mindful. But with modern life, and its myriad modern distractions, we are un-learning this innate ability. We're de-skilling. We're losing the power and wonder of our naturally mindful minds.

One simple way to access this kind of mood state is with simple breathing exercises. We usually breathe unconsciously, but if we take the trouble to direct our conscious focus towards our breathing, it can have profound effects. When your out-breath is longer than your in-breath, you activate the parasympathetic nervous system, which you can think of as your relaxation mode. The opposite of this is our sympathetic nervous system, which is our fight-or-flight mode. Many of us spend too much time in fight-or-flight mode, and not enough in relaxation mode.

3–4–5 BREATHING

I've come up with a simple exercise called 3–4–5 breathing. It couldn't be easier. Just breathe in for three seconds, hold for four and then breathe out for five. It's easy to remember and even easier to do.

I remember one patient, forty-eight-year-old Brian, who worked in a stressful job in a bank. Every lunch break he would furiously puff away on cigarettes for twenty minutes to try and relieve his stress. He felt anxious returning to work after lunch and this would last all the way through the evening, well after finishing work. This had deleterious effects on his sleep. I suggested that he try 3–4–5 breathing

every lunchtime. This was quite an alien concept to Brian, but he agreed to give it a go. He only did it for a few minutes in his car every lunchtime but the benefits were immediate. At my next consultation he reported reduced stress, reduced anxiety, better focus throughout the afternoon and, incredibly, better sleep at night. All from consciously changing his breathing at lunchtime. Having felt the benefits, those few minutes became longer and longer, and now he does fifteen minutes every day. Brian started small and built up big. You can too. The important thing is just to start.

Even two minutes per day will have benefits. Not got two minutes? Really? Do you manage to brush your teeth morning and night? I suspect you do. Why? Because it has been prioritized since childhood and that priority has now become a routine. Perhaps it is time to create a new routine: two minutes of conscious breathing per day. Try to do this at the same time every day – it is much more likely to become a habit if you do.

One of the main problems I find when talking about these ideas to patients is that people assume they can't do it. I've yet to find a patient for whom this is actually true, *once they've found the right form of stillness practice for them*. Another problem is giving up too soon. Patients often say, 'Doctor, I tried it twice, I just couldn't do it.' But I ask them, 'If I asked you to run the London marathon, would you try to run twenty-six miles two or three times and then say "I can't do it", or would you build up gradually?' Most people understand that, to complete a marathon, you have to train your body to do it. In the same way, you have to train your mind to get used to practising stillness.

If you prefer to sit cross-legged on a special stool chanting 'Om' or staring into a candle, that's fine – but there is no right or wrong way to do it. There are a million ways to meditate and one of them will suit you. You can meditate whilst walking, if you're present as you're doing it. Try focusing on your walking next time you are out. Focus on your feet hitting the ground. Be aware of the trees swaying in the breeze. Be mindful and pay attention. It is a completely different experience from walking whilst texting, sending emails and checking your social media feed.

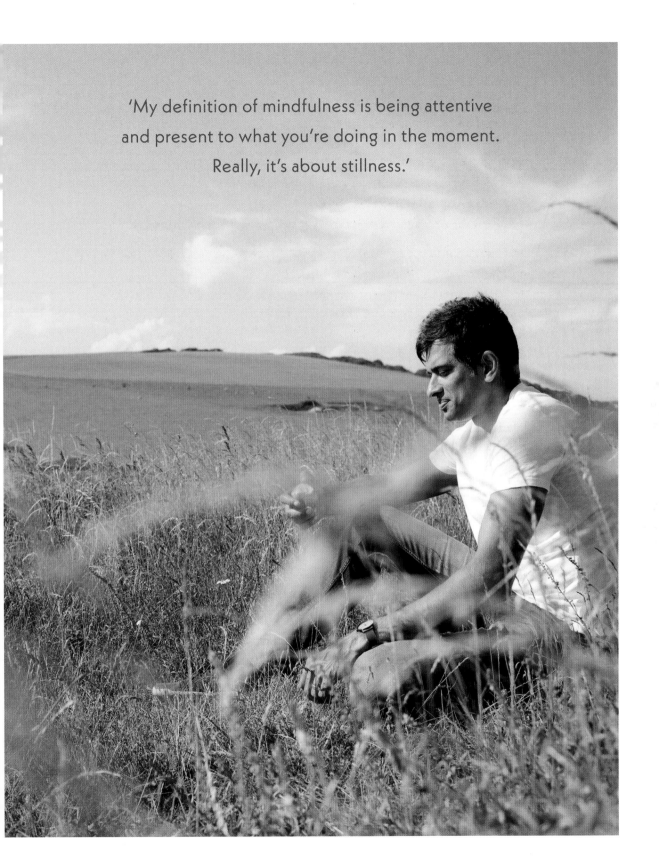

'My definition of mindfulness is being attentive
and present to what you're doing in the moment.
Really, it's about stillness.'

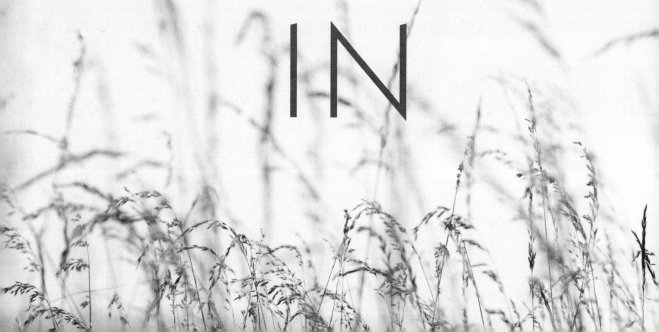

JUST
BREATHE
IN

FOR THREE SECONDS,

HOLD

FOR

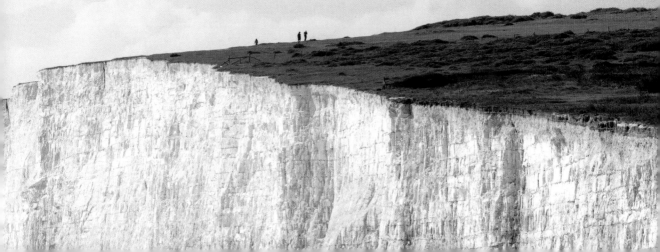

FOUR

AND

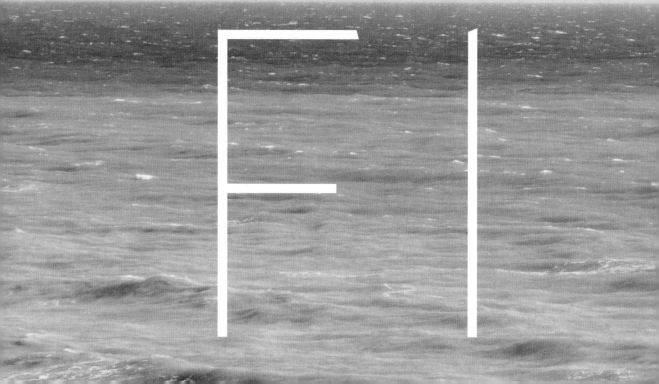

THEN

BREATHE

FI

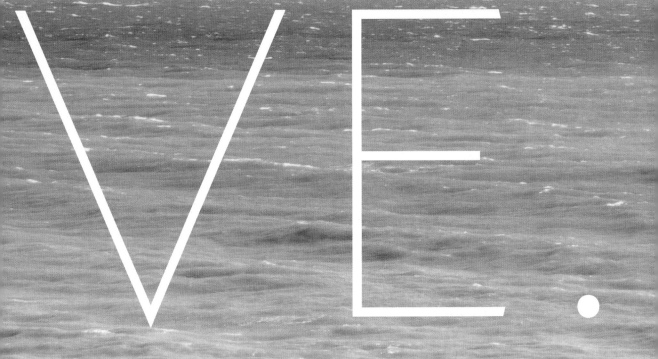

OUT FOR

VE.

Tai Chi is a form of moving meditation. You could do what Brian did and practise 3–4–5 breathing during your lunch break. You could do what I did and download an app that gives guided meditation (I recommend Calm or Headspace). What I like about apps is they help me feel like I'm *doing* something. You plug in your headphones and you press play. *I am doing something now!* Then you follow the spoken instructions. My wife, on the other hand, can't stand them – she is able to switch off, so finds it irritating to have a voice talking to her whilst she is meditating. And that's fine. Just do whatever works for you. You don't even have to use the same method every time. Mix it up!

There really are no rules. Pick something you like and start doing it, even for a few minutes every day. You can do it wherever you want. In bed first thing in the morning or even last thing at night before you go to sleep. In the car at lunchtime. How about mindful cooking where you are completely lost in what you are doing?

Another common obstacle to success is self-judgement. If you find it hard, don't judge yourself. I tried Tai Chi for the first time as part of a BBC documentary series I was filming and found it impossibly difficult. The instructor (known as the sensei) kept telling me to relax but I just couldn't seem to get my head round it. Most of us haven't been mindful in years, so we shouldn't immediately expect to feel like the Dalai Lama. Don't be harsh on yourself. If your thoughts are racing, let them race, that's OK – just make sure that you're observing them as they do it. That's still one step better than yesterday, when you didn't know your thoughts were racing and you were just being carried along in the relentless stampede.

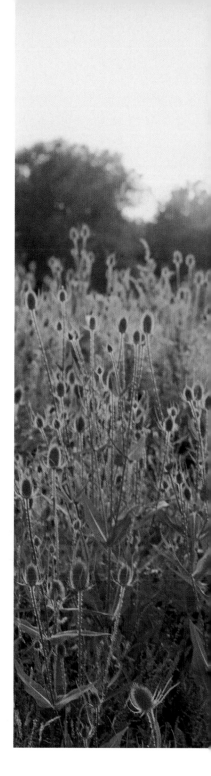

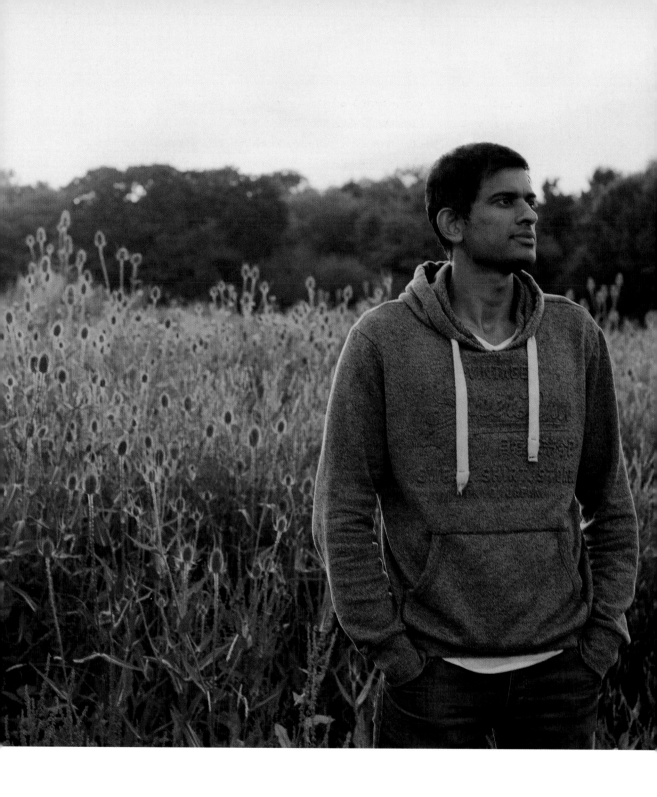

Many of our natural capacities for stillness are lost as we grow into adults, and all the pressures and responsibilities of real life kick in. That's why it can be instructive to look at kids. They don't multitask; they focus on what they're doing. When I watch my son playing, he sometimes can't even hear what I'm saying, he's so focused on his latest Lego creation. If my daughter is painting a picture, I may as well be invisible – she is completely immersed in the process. It's the same as when Tiger Woods was playing well and dominating the golf world. Someone like that, fully involved in the match, doesn't hear the crowds. He doesn't even *see* the crowds. He's in the zone. In a very real way, he's practising mindfulness. He's utterly present, there in the moment. This is sometimes known to psychologists as 'flow state'.

ACHIEVING FLOW

Flow does not need to be the preserve of high-performing athletes or Buddhist monks. We can all experience our own flow state – but we need to find out what it is that puts us into it, because it's different for everyone. We also need to be strict about scheduling time for it and making sure we're not disturbed, otherwise we'll never get there. I'm as prone as anyone to the distractions of the modern world. Even whilst writing this book, I've found myself constantly distracted by text messages, phone calls, mindless surfing and quick peeks at Facebook. I only managed to complete it by switching off my phone. It can be helpful to use apps (I recommend Freedom and Anti-Social, which are available at freedom.to and antisocial.80pct.com) to block the internet. But I've also experienced flow state on many occasions. I'm a keen musician and have spent a lot of my life writing and performing. When I'm working on a new song, I can become utterly lost in my own creative process. When cutting tracks at the studio, it's not uncommon for eight hours to pass like eight minutes. Why? Because I'm in flow! Time passes in a different way because I have complete immersion in what I'm doing. This is a form of stillness. The stresses and distractions of ordinary life are blocked and the mind is in a peak state of focus.

The growing awareness that many of us are losing this skill has led to the popularity of adult colouring books. It's remarkable how still your mind has to be to engage with colouring-in and perhaps this will be the first entry point for you. If you're more familiar with yoga, you might have heard of the sequence called Surya Namaskar or sun salutation. This is a series of postures that incorporate controlled movements and breathing. Five minutes of focused sun salutations, if done mindfully, can be fantastically restorative and help you fully rejuvenate. There are many different options for your five-minute practice of stillness. The more you practise, the easier you'll find it becomes. Even better, as your five-minute daily practice becomes ingrained as a new habit, you'll find this will help you to be more mindful when engaging in your fifteen minutes of me-time at the top of this pillar.

If you're not lucky enough to be able to completely immerse yourself in your favourite pastime for five minutes or more every day, then practise stillness wherever you can: in the car, in a coffee shop . . . you can even do it in the fitting room of a clothes shop. If you have the smartphone app and some headphones, you can do it more or less anywhere. On many occasions, I have done mine on the train. A great tip is to do it at the same time every day. That way, it becomes a habit, and if you consciously change your habits, you unconsciously change your biology. These are the little daily decisions that work on your body in the same way as medicine. If there was a drug that could do what regular stillness practice can do, it would be worth billions. It really is that powerful.

Ideally, you should aim to build up to ten or fifteen minutes per day. But you don't need to start there. Begin slowly if you need to. Even two minutes is a good start. It can be intimidating if you have never done it before and we cannot expect that, after years of having an overactive monkey-mind, we will immediately be able to switch it off.

When was the last time you were fully immersed in something you loved? What gives you that flow? Is it gardening? Reading? Cooking? Painting? Tinkering with engines? Whatever it is, seize it. Own it. Guard it. Practise it. Use it as your way of gaining stillness.

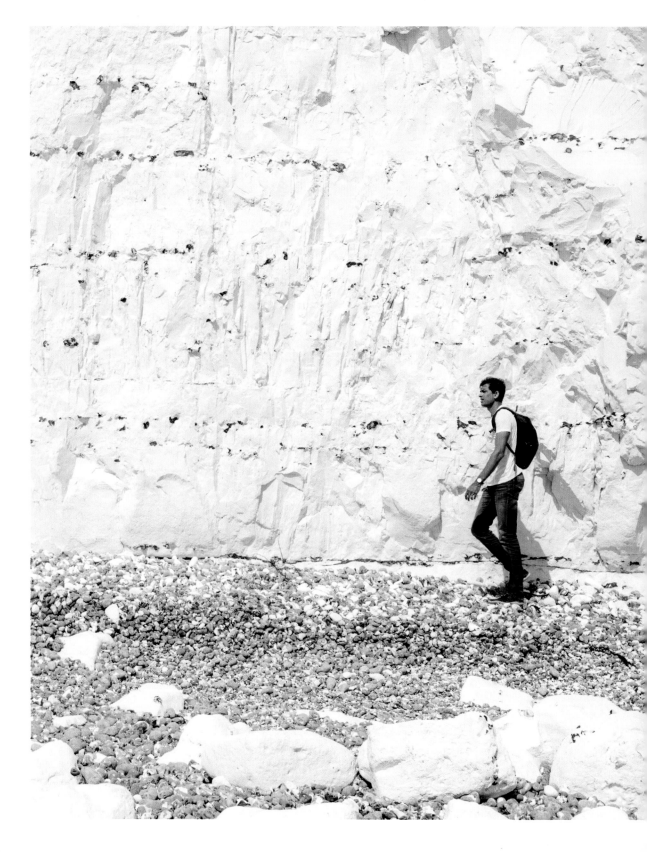

STILLNESS INTERVENTIONS YOU
MIGHT THINK OF TRYING:

To get a tick in this section requires dedicated daily introspective practice, and so my top recommendations would be meditation (guided or unguided), or deep breathing.

Meditation with an app like Calm

Deep breathing

Yoga breathing practices such as breathing in through left nostril for four, holding for four, and breathing out through the right

3–4–5 breathing

Five minutes of colouring-in

Sitting in silence with full awareness of your senses, e.g. feel your feet on the floor, the breeze on your cheeks etc.

Listening to music mindfully – headphones on, eyes closed, fully focused

5. RECLAIM YOUR DINING TABLE

Eat one meal a day at the table, in company (if possible), without your devices.

When I was a child, Mum would always take the time to make us home-cooked meals. My parents were raised in Kolkata and this was just part of the lifestyle there. Pretty much everyone in India cooked from scratch. But growing up in the 1980s, in the north of England, I had no idea how lucky I was. Mum would prepare piles and piles of sizzling, fragrant, delicious food and there would always be containers of it stacked in the fridge in perfect portion-sized Tupperware boxes. If I was ever hungry, I could just raid the fridge, dish some food out onto a plate and warm it up in the microwave. My favourite was chicken curry with rice. I remember pacing impatiently up and down, waiting for the oven to ping, before perching myself on a chair at the breakfast bar to blow on forkfuls of rich, sweet, spicy curry and shovelling it, still scorching hot, into my mouth. It was heaven.

But as I got older, and there was more exam pressure from school, this slowly but surely developed into a bad habit. And not just for me. My brothers and I would come home from school and our plates would get warmed up one at a time in a microwave; then we'd each carry our meals with burning fingertips to be eaten separately on the sofa in front of *Neighbours*. I can see why my folks thought they were doing us a favour. If we caught up on our favourite Australian soaps whilst we were eating, that left more time later on for homework! And they were right, we did gain valuable study time. But we lost something else – something that I believe today is perhaps even more important. What we lost was that feeling of us all sitting around together, gossiping, laughing, bickering and doing all the things a family should be doing when they get together. What we lost was connection.

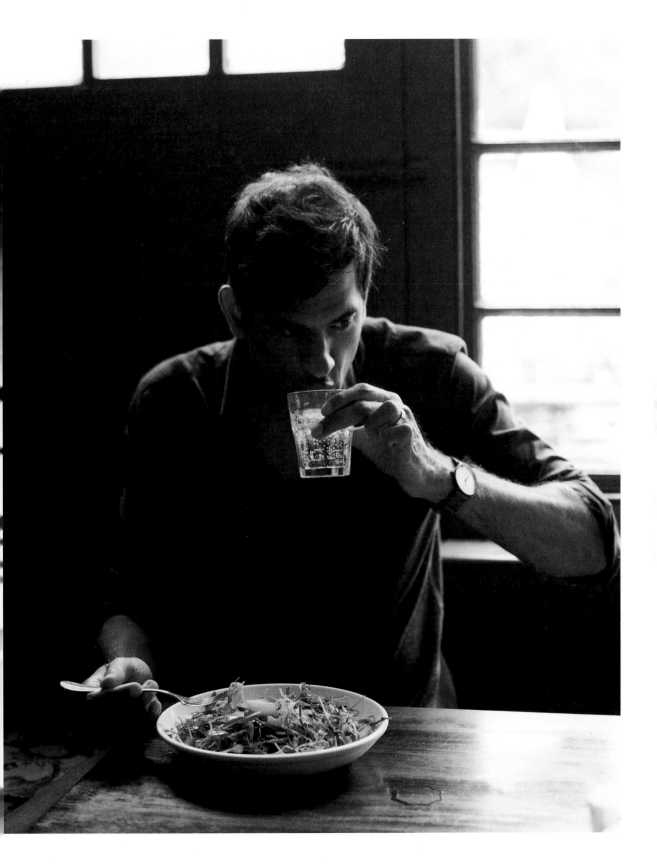

FIRELIGHT TALK

All those hundreds of thousands of years ago, when the design of our bodies was still being developed by the slow forces of evolution, I suspect we never went off to eat by ourselves like this. And it isn't just common sense that tells me so. It's actually possible to get a decent idea of what life was like when we existed in hunter-gatherer tribes because there are many still in existence, in parts of the world that have had little contact with modernity. One of these tribes, the Ju/'hoansi bushmen, lives in Namibia. Researchers who study their behaviour report fascinating switches at different times of the day. During daylight hours, their conversation is mostly devoted to practical outcomes such as possible hunting strategies and the mediation of arguments. But, when the sun goes down, all that changes. Around the campfire, more than 81 per cent of their conversation time is spent telling each other stories. The researchers call this 'firelight talk'. It's a time of calmness, reflection and – perhaps most importantly – connection.

It's only in the last few years that the importance of social connection to physical health has started to become clear. Because we've evolved as tribal creatures, living happily in large groups, the brain interprets social isolation as a major problem. Once again, in this situation the body thinks it's under attack and puts itself in a kind of emergency mode. Levels of the stress hormone cortisol tend to be higher in lonely people. There's also evidence it triggers our fight-or-flight stress response, causing chronic inflammation to increase. One major meta-analysis from 2012 that collected data from over 100,000 people found the effects of feeling socially unconnected were comparable to smoking and roughly three times more damaging to health than being obese. Another study that followed the effects of loneliness over time found that feeling isolated in 2002 was predictive of who'd be dead just six years later. Loneliness expert Professor John Cacioppo compares the state to pain, hunger and thirst. 'You would not want to be in these states, at least not for very long,' he says, 'but each has evolved as an aversive biological signal that motivates us to do something that's good for us. Physical pain motivates us to take care of our physical body. Loneliness motivates us to take care of our social body.'

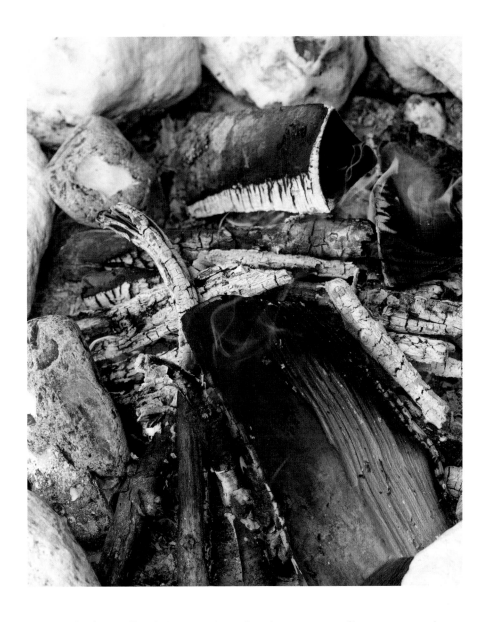

'Firelight talk'. It's a time of calmness, reflection and –
perhaps most importantly – connection.

RECLAIMING YOUR DINING TABLE

This is why I recommend eating at a table. I know that the Ju/'hoansi aren't doing this, but the point of this intervention is not the furniture, it's the togetherness. In the modern West, the table rather than the campfire is where our connection, or our 'firelight talk', happens. And that's not the only benefit it brings. Sitting helps take us out of fight-or-flight mode and puts us into relaxation mode, by activating the parasympathetic nervous system (see page 25). You digest food properly when you're in relaxation mode. When you're in fight-or-flight, you don't. Eating at the table also means we're likely to consume less. Recent research from academics at the University of Birmingham has found that when we eat in front of the television not only do we consume more at that particular meal, we also take in more calories later in the day.

Why is this? It might surprise you to learn that hunger isn't the only thing that affects how much you eat – memory also plays a part. If we're absorbed with watching a cheetah chasing an antelope on the latest David Attenborough documentary whilst mindlessly shovelling food into our mouths, we'll probably remember less of our meal, and may start getting 'I'm hungry' signals sooner. Attention also plays a role, and for similar reasons. After around twenty minutes of eating, the brain starts sending its 'I'm full' signals. These signals are partly dependent on how much we've already eaten – information that comes not only from the sheer volume of food we've swallowed, but also how much of it we've seen, smelled and tasted.

Even as recently as twenty years ago it was common for families to eat their evening meals together. Nearly every house – even smaller ones – had a space reserved for doing exactly that. Nowadays, some homes don't even contain a dining table. Communal eating has been a basic part of the human condition for hundreds of thousands of years and yet over the last few decades it's almost completely vanished from many British households. Our dining rooms have been knocked through, often to make even bigger spaces in which to watch TV. But this doesn't have to continue; the good news is that it's an easy problem to fix. There are many different options to suit all budgets, including foldaway tables if space is limited.

Recently, Jenny and Paul, a couple I see at my practice, started to make a point of eating together at my suggestion. Jenny, who is fifty-one, has always struggled with her weight and suffers from mood swings. Her husband Paul, who is fifty-two, meanwhile, doesn't sleep well and has a daily two-hour commute to and from work. He's constantly tired and is starting to lay down fat around his middle. Just five years ago, this guy was in tip-top shape.

After just one week of sitting and eating together, and moving from a processed diet to a wholefood diet, they told me they felt like completely different people. Now they're talking more, they're finding out about each other's day, they're more mindful about what and how much they're eating. Of course, I don't know whether it's the eating together or the better diet that's having the greater effect – and, in truth, it doesn't really matter. The point is, it's about the threshold. These two interventions have moved them in the right direction, back towards the right side of their personal thresholds. They're eating better, they're eating less and they're feeling closer. These changes alone are having profoundly positive effects.

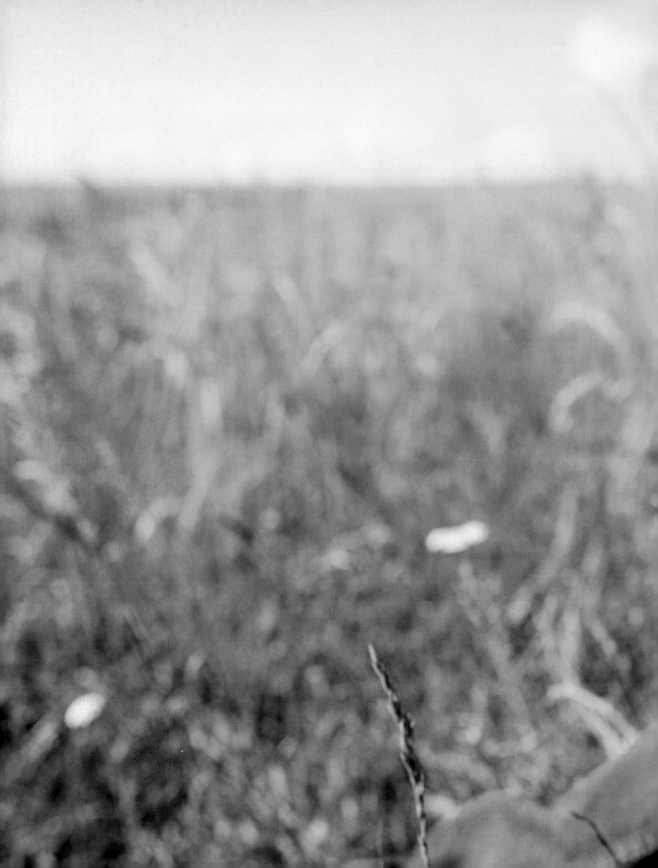

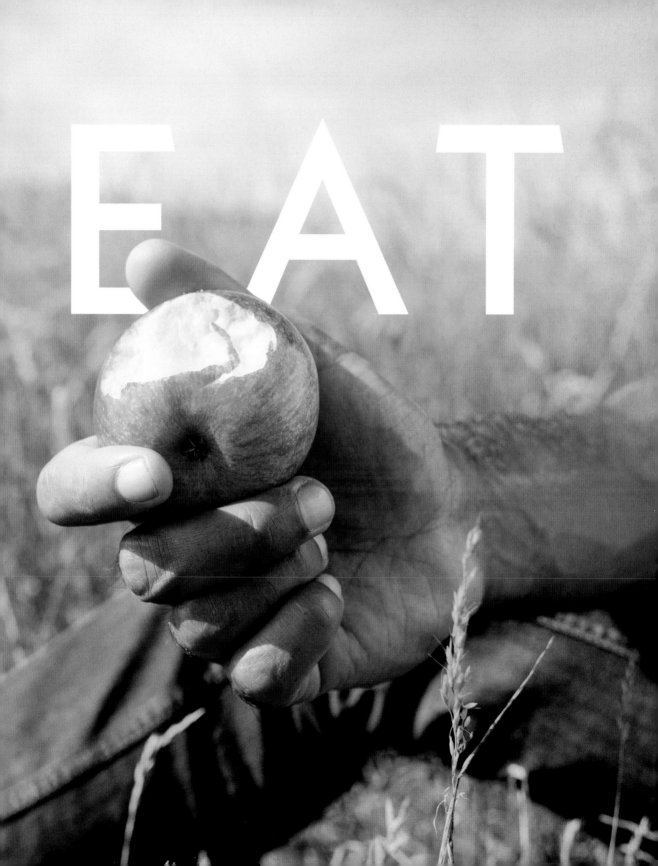

Perhaps because we live in a culture that's obsessed with appearance, we've become dangerously caught up in thinking that diet is merely about weight. It's forced us to focus relentlessly on fats and carbs. Many of us, especially those over the age of thirty, have grown up being told that we should eat a low-fat diet. It's only recently become clear that such advice was at least partly misguided, and it's led to some unfortunate and unintended consequences. In practice, cutting out the fat often meant ramping up the sugar and refined and heavily processed carbohydrates, with all too predictable results. We also forgot that fat – as long as it's the right kind – can be good for you.

But this doesn't mean we should make the same mistake again by going too far and deciding that it's all about eating a high-fat diet. There's always a tendency to overcorrect and oversimplify. It's tempting to believe that there is, somewhere out there, the perfect diet and all we need to do to achieve perfect health is find it. Many people, of course, believe they've already done so: low-fat, high-fat, high-protein, low-carb, vegetarian, vegan, the list goes on. And it's true that each of these options will be effective for some people, but none is a one-size-fits-all solution.

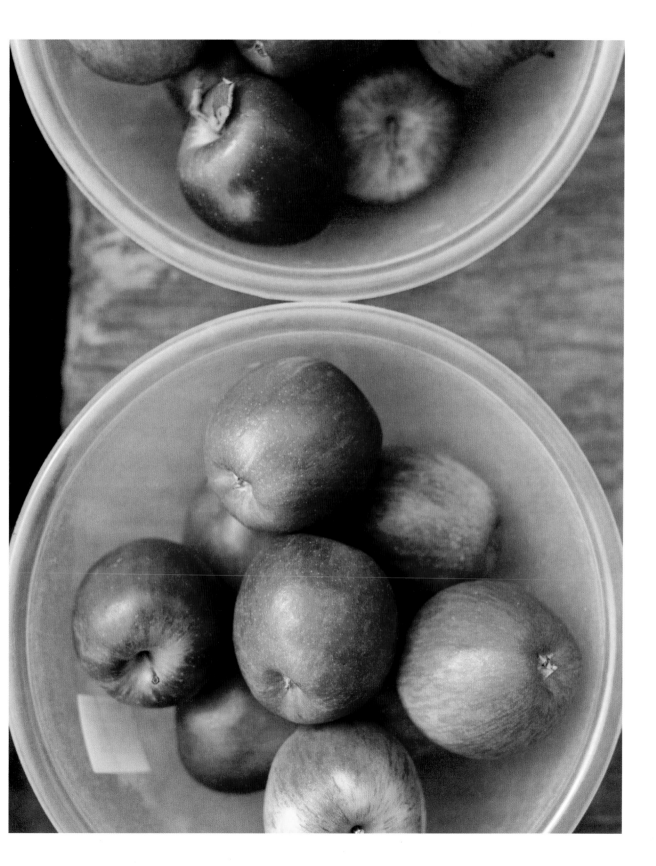

A huge problem with today's food culture is the sheer amount of conflicting advice that's flying about the place. Contrary to what you might think, I don't necessarily have a problem with any of it. If being a vegan or sticking to your own interpretation of 'paleo' is working for you, that's fantastic. But I simply refuse to believe there's One True Diet that's optimal for everyone. Remember, humans have always been opportunistic omnivores. All through history our diets have been dictated by geography and climate. We ate whatever food was available. This means the evolved human machine is capable of thriving on a whole range of diets.

BLUE-ZONE DIETS

Around the world, there are some apparently almost magical enclaves where the proportion of people who live past 100 is up to ten times higher than the average rate. They are nearly always in good health, with much lower rates of chronic degenerative diseases such as dementia, heart attacks and strokes. These places have been coined 'blue zones' by the Belgian scientist Michel Poulain. As you might imagine, blue zones have been widely studied by nutritional scientists hoping to discover the One True Diet. And what do you think they found? That the secret of blue zones was low carb? Vegetarian? Gluten free? Not a bit of it. What they actually found was an enormous variety of diets. Some were eating meat; some, like the Seventh Day Adventists in California, were vegetarians; some were eating more fish whilst others, like the Okinawans, were feasting on high-carb foods like sweet potatoes.

WHAT IS THE RIGHT DIET FOR YOU?

One drawback to giving generalized food advice is that the correct diet for any individual really depends on their state of health. Someone who has been abusing their body for twenty years will have to make more dietary changes to get to the same place as someone who's in relatively good shape. The optimal diet for you is likely to evolve and change as you grow older. A child will usually have different health priorities from those of an octogenarian, just as a bodybuilder will, compared to an expectant mother.

Having said all that, there do appear to be some very broad and basic principles that are consistent among all the blue-zone diets:

- None has a processed-food culture. By and large, they eat fresh, unprocessed, local produce.

- They all sit down and eat meals together.

- They eat what's in season.

- They have treats, but only at very special festival times such as Christmas and Easter, not every day after school, or every Friday or Saturday.

It is these principles that I intend to focus on.

MAKING A CHANGE

There are five suggested interventions for this pillar. Each one will help you improve your health, and the good news is that they all connect with each other, so when you start doing one, the other four become considerably easier. They are applicable to everyone, no matter what your dietary preference: meat eater, pescetarian, vegetarian or vegan.

They are designed to be sustainable and achievable and you should take them at your own pace. For those of you who what more direction, I would suggest starting with 'De-normalize sugar' and 'Daily micro-fasts'. These can rapidly improve the way you feel and make it significantly easier to achieve the other interventions.

A SPECIAL WORD ON GLUTEN AND DAIRY

Although not a specific part of *The Four Pillar Plan* I'd like to share with you an intervention that I have seen change many patients lives – elimination diets. These diets are hotly debated and are surrounded by a lot of confusion and emotion. Here's my perspective.

GOING GLUTEN FREE

Humans have evolved eating whatever was available, typically meat, fish, eggs, vegetables, fruit, nuts, seeds and legumes. It appears that grains such as wheat and barley are relatively new introductions, but that doesn't mean we haven't evolved to eat them. Unlike some experts, I'm not completely anti-grain, but when I want to treat a patient with a specific problem such as joint pain, headaches or eczema, I'll often ask them to avoid gluten-containing grains for a four-week period. That means cutting out things like bread, pasta and cereals. Many people react to these foods without realizing it, and removing them from one's diet can reduce inflammation.

CUTTING OUT DAIRY

It's the same with dairy. Some people appear to tolerate dairy just fine and may derive health benefits from consuming it, but for many it causes adverse effects. At least 75 per cent of the world's population are thought to be intolerant to lactose, a sugar present in milk and cheese (yoghurt tends to have much lower amounts). That number will be significantly lower in the UK as the problem is more prevalent among certain ethnicities, such as those from Asia and Africa, but even if you're not lactose intolerant, a significant number of Britons have a sensitivity to different components in dairy, such as the protein casein.

Many patients I see have spent their lives entirely unaware that they're unable to process it properly and are amazed when symptoms they've lived with for years suddenly clear up. A recent patient of mine had spent years suffering from severe heartburn and a longstanding dry cough. Despite multiple medications, dozens of specialist appointments and four invasive endoscopic investigations, his daily life was unbearable. After three weeks on an elimination diet, his problems cleared up entirely. He tried reintroducing the eliminated foods and his symptoms returned. He didn't need me to convince him. He was sold. He remains symptom-free to this day.

I've seen complaints such as recurrent sinus or tonsil infections, skin conditions such as eczema, migraines, IBS and heartburn, mucus production and problematic mood changes disappear when patients eliminate these foods. That said, I never recommend the 'gluten-free' products found on retailers' shelves, many of which are highly processed and full of sugar. I recommend instead whole foods which naturally do not contain gluten, such as meat, fish, fruit, vegetables, rice and buckwheat. There's a false perception that giving up gluten is necessary only for sufferers of coeliac disease. A plethora of studies have shown this not to be the case.

Misguided commentators in the media have portrayed the avoidance of gluten, and dairy, as some sort of dietary fad, as if they are somehow essential food groups. They are not. There are several populations around the world who consume little to no dairy, such as the Chinese, and do just fine.

Medical practitioners tend to require hard evidence that a certain food is causing an issue before asking a patient to try cutting it out. The problem with that approach is that such proof is often hard to get, with even blood tests being notoriously unreliable. I'm not convinced we should demand such rigour before giving it a go. A well-managed elimination diet is both free and harmless while potentially resulting in a vast improvement to your health.

It can be helpful to get professional advice to help structure your own elimination diet to ensure you are consuming your full spectrum of nutrients.

1. DE-NORMALIZE SUGAR

Retrain your taste buds by removing all sugars from your cupboards and get into the habit of always reading the label on your food to check the sugar content.

This has been one of the hardest chapters for me to write. Why? Because sugar is absolutely everywhere these days, and hides where you least expect it. All of my patients consume wildly different amounts of sugar but what is consistent, amongst pretty much all of them, is that they are consuming too much – at least, with respect to their health. My goal with this particular intervention is to help you reset your relationship with sugar. The best way to do this is to dramatically reduce your consumption, but to do that, you first need to know where the sugar is.

We have outsourced our food choices to massive global corporations. They're deciding what goes into their products and, therefore, what goes on in our bodies. In this way, decisions made in faraway corporate boardrooms are causing cascades of biological changes to happen inside us – changes that could cause pain, stress, infirmity and even shorten our lives. This might sound melodramatic but it is, nevertheless, unarguably true.

Take sugar. If you're eating processed or pre-packed food there's a very good chance that your intake of the sticky white stuff is through the roof. The only way to get any real idea about the amount you're consuming is to get into the habit of looking at labels. I'm still mesmerized by how many seemingly healthy packaged foods have sugar as a prominent ingredient. If you go into a branch of one popular high-street supermarket, you can pick up packs of sliced roast chicken breast from the chiller cabinet that contain sugar.

Why does meat need sugar in it? Please tell me. I'm asking because I genuinely don't know. These retailers are playing fast and loose with our health – and our National Health Service – simply to gain the very tiniest imagined advantage over their rivals. Sugar is finding its way into more and more of our foodstuffs, and it's we who end up paying, not only at the tills but also with our health. Type 2 diabetes is now at genuine crisis levels in the UK. Since 1996 the number of Britons diagnosed with the condition has more than doubled, from 1.4 million to nearly 3.5 million. On top of that, there's an estimated further 1.1 million currently living with it, undiagnosed. An extraordinary £10 billion – 10 per cent of the NHS's entire budget – is spent treating it annually. That's £27 million every single day. More than £1 million an hour. Even the food we give our children is spiked with sugar. The recommended daily intake limit for children is five cubes and the average British child consumes three cubes at breakfast alone!

One of the most troubling trends I've seen over my sixteen years of practice as a doctor is an increasing number of children who refuse to eat fruit or vegetables at all. On an evolutionary level, when has this ever happened? It's truly bizarre. But it's a measure of the extent to which the food industry has hijacked our bodies. We should feel outraged by this. A peach used to be a delicious summer treat, but if your taste buds have grown used to Haribo, something as beautiful and wonderful as a perfectly ripe peach rapidly loses its magic. We are allowing these corporations to blunt our own inbuilt, *proper* taste perceptions.

CHANGING YOUR TASTE BUDS

A part of the problem is that overconsumption of sugar seems to alter our taste buds. As they become used to it, our bodies crave more and more. One illuminating 2016 study compared two groups of people who, initially, were consuming the same amount of sugar. One group was put on a low-sugar diet whilst the other group continued on their existing one. The group consuming a low-sugar diet rated the same dessert as sweeter than the group who had not reduced their sugar intake. As every month passed, they rated it as more and more sweet. This is further evidence that reducing your intake of sugar changes your sense of taste. This certainly mirrors my own experience as well as that of my patients. Many years ago, I used to have sugar in my tea. When I first tried it without, the taste was disgusting. But fast forward a few weeks, I accidentally picked up someone else's sugared tea at work and almost spat it out.

One of the major issues is that we're biologically hard wired to crave sugar. One of the world's leading experts in evolutionary biology, Harvard's Professor Daniel Lieberman, says that sugar is a 'deep, ancient craving' that probably evolved to help us survive. Gorging on sweet fruits during the summer enabled us to store fat that we then used during periods of food scarcity in the winter. 'Simply put,' Lieberman has said, 'humans evolved to crave sugar, store it and then use it. For millions of years, our cravings and digestive systems were exquisitely balanced because sugar was rare. Apart from honey, most of the foods our hunter-gatherer ancestors ate were no sweeter than a carrot.' We're wired to crave sugar in order to store it as energy in the form of fat. But modern food technology has allowed ultra-sweet flavours to proliferate. A once useful survival adaptation has now become problematic.

Because there's so much sugar in our diets, we continually find our blood sugar levels soaring. Studies into the effects of these sudden sugar spikes on the brain have found they trigger intense activation in a region called the nucleus accumbens, an area that's involved with reward, pleasure, addiction and saliency (how drawn you are to a stimulus that causes these effects, such as a chocolate bar or a milkshake). Remarkably, this is the same area that lights up in people who have addictions to drugs such as cocaine, heroin and nicotine. Our consumption of high-sugar foods is having a similar impact on the brain. Some researchers believe we can't say that food is addictive in the same way as cocaine because we need food to live. But I say we do not need sugar to live. For me, it's absolutely clear sugar has genuinely addictive properties.

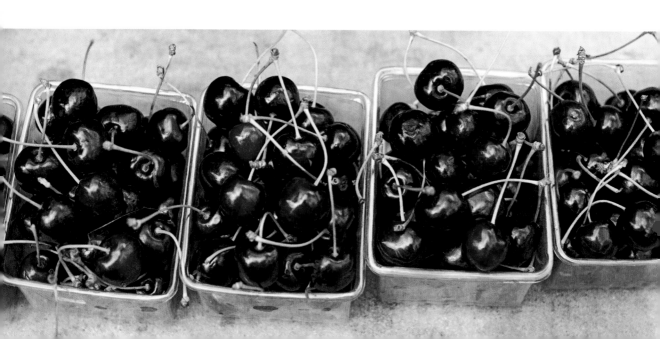

SYMPTOMS THAT MAY INDICATE
OVERRELIANCE ON SUGAR:

Feeling the need to eat every two hours

Concentration dropping mid-morning

Experiencing an afternoon slump

Feeling hungry – irritability between meals

Feeling shaky or dizzy

Experiencing a huge boost in energy or fatigue after your meal

Overreliance on caffeine and sugar to 'keep me going'

Craving for sweet foods and snacks between meals

Feeling light-headed if you're late for a meal

Our unrelenting consumption of sugar, whether it's an obvious component of a bag of sweets or hidden way down the ingredients list in our supermarket wholemeal bread, sets us off on a blood-sugar rollercoaster. If you start the day with foods that are either high in sugar or are converted in your body to sugar (foods like white bread and breakfast cereal), your blood sugar soars and you go into a buzzy high. Two to three hours later, however, it crashes. Then you're craving sugar again. My patients always tell me, 'I need to eat every few hours because, when I don't, I get shaky and I really need something.' That's a symptom. It shows me they're probably riding that sugary rollercoaster. If humans really did have an inability to go more than a few hours without food, we'd have died out long ago. The fix isn't to keep feeding the rollercoaster, it's to get off it completely.

YOUR DIABETES RISK

If we don't get our sugar consumption managed properly, there's a serious risk we're going to end up damaging our health. There's a strong likelihood we could even end up with type 2 diabetes. The important thing to know about this disease is that by the time you end up with a diagnosis, things will have been going wrong in your body for many years already. It's not something like a chest infection, in that you have it or you don't.

The formal diagnosis comes only when you pass a certain arbitrary point along a scale. This, in a nutshell, is how it works. One of the body's key functions is to keep blood sugar within a tightly controlled range. When you consume sugar or foods that are quickly converted to sugar, such as most supermarket bread and bagels, your body pumps out a tiny dose of a hormone called insulin to bring your levels back to normal. The problem is, if we've been abusing this system for a long period of time, our bodies become resistant to this tiny dose of insulin, needing more and more of it to have the same effect. In high amounts, insulin is toxic. Your body is now poisoning itself. When this poisoning gets to a certain level and your blood sugar can no longer be adequately controlled, we call it 'diabetes'. But that's just the end stage of a long process that's been going on for years.

TYPE 2 DIABETES

There are many factors, in addition to excessive sugar consumption, that contribute to the development of insulin resistance and type 2 diabetes. They include:

- Too much highly processed food

- Physical inactivity and low muscle mass

- Sleep deprivation

- Persistently high stress levels

- Disturbed gut bug ecosystem (see page 98)

- Low levels of vitamin D, usually caused by lack of sunshine

- Environmental toxins

Many patients will have more than one contributory factor, which is why a 360-degree approach to health such as the one outlined in this book is so important.

If a diagnosis of type 2 diabetes has already been made, there are some special dietary considerations that should be followed. Diabetics have a relatively low tolerance of carbohydrates, particularly refined carbohydrates. This is why I advise those affected to reduce their intake of all refined and processed carbohydrates such as bread, pasta, bagels and muffins, and even non-refined ones like white potatoes that can also spike your blood sugar. In the short term I also advise them to eat fewer starchy vegetables such as sweet potatoes, parsnips and carrots whilst I address the underlying causes. I always aim to reintroduce these starchy vegetables at a later date owing to their beneficial impact on the gut microbiome, though that isn't always possible without a detrimental effect. I have also found that periods of fasting can be very helpful in reducing insulin and sugar levels.

Note – if you are type 2 diabetic and on medication, you must consult a healthcare professional before making significant changes to your diet such as prolonged fasting.

BEYOND DIABETES

A great many of us, after years of gorging sugar and junk, have unknowingly become insulin resistant. On top of the 3.5 million Britons who are thought to have passed the point of a full diagnosis, an incredible one in three adults in Britain are thought to have what's known as 'pre-diabetes'. This means they're already insulin resistant, to a certain degree. They're being poisoned, they just don't yet realize it.

But sugar's doing more than just giving us type 2 diabetes. As we have just learned, sugar increases our insulin levels and one of insulin's main roles is to direct fat storage. It tells our bodies to hold on to fat by storing it, so more insulin means we're heavier. Chronically raised insulin levels have been associated with:

- Obesity

- Increased levels of VLDL – a particularly harmful form of cholesterol

- Raised blood pressure owing to increased retention of salt and water

- Increased breast cancer risk

- Raised testosterone levels in women, which is associated with conditions such as polycystic ovaries

But, as bad as all this might sound, it's important that we don't swing too far in the other direction. I don't buy the hypothesis that sugar alone is responsible for the obesity epidemic. It is a big contributor, sure, but it isn't the whole story. Obesity, and any chronic manifestation of suboptimal health, has many contributing factors and that's why this programme is focused on balancing all aspects of health.

Good, sustainable health isn't about demonizing any one aspect of our diets – whether it's fat, carbs or even sugar. Humans have been eating honey for hundreds of thousands of years. The point is, it should be an occasional treat rather than the daily norm.

TAKING THE PLUNGE

Some of my patients prefer to go 'cold turkey' and cut out all sugar for fourteen days. This can be an excellent way to retrain your taste buds quickly, but will often lead to withdrawal symptoms such as headaches, irritability and insomnia, especially between days 3 and 6. However, once past ten days, patients often report many benefits, including improved sleep, mood and energy.

You might prefer a more gradual reduction in your sugar intake. This is absolutely fine. You should go at a pace that you are comfortable with. Cutting it out of your tea is a great place to start – that's what I did. No matter where you start from, reducing your sugar intake will benefit your health.

Whichever route you choose, you will have to start training yourself to look at ingredient lists. Sugar is lurking where you least expect it, and in many different disguises such as glucose, dextrose, glucose syrup, cane sugar, glucose-fructose syrup, molasses, cane juice and rice syrup. Whilst you are retraining your taste buds, I would also recommend you avoid 'natural' forms of sugar such as honey and maple syrup.

Try to purge your house of all sugars, both hidden and obvious. We all crave sugar. So what do you think's going to happen when you come home after a bad day at work, stressed out? If that packet of biscuits or chocolate is sitting in the cupboard, do you really think willpower will be enough? Every day, every week, every month? Hell, no! You *will* crack.

INCREASE YOUR CHANCES OF SUCCESS

However you approach cutting down your sugar intake, you might find the following strategies helpful:

- **Plan limited social engagements for the first two weeks;** these are the hardest times when cutting out or reducing sugar intake. Being around other people, and their chocolate and puddings, can be a big source of temptation

- **Keep healthy snacks readily available at home, at work, and even in the car** – carrots and hummus, celery and nut butter, a piece of fruit or some olives. One of my patients used to take boiled eggs into work, which she would eat any time she felt peckish

- **Remove artificial sweeteners;** you need to retrain your taste buds, and artificial sweeteners will sabotage that process by maintaining your damaged sense of what sweetness really is

- **Include some protein in every meal:** meat, fish, eggs, nuts and/or seeds; protein keeps you feeling full for longer, which helps avoid sugar cravings

- **Be prepared – get into the habit of keeping emergency snacks with you;** when travelling, I will take with me a can of wild salmon and some nuts and seeds, which help me to resist temptation when out, hungry and surrounded by sweet scents and alluring packets

Once you have reset your relationship with sugar, you can begin to consume it *intentionally*.

Take back control of your taste buds and tune in to your body's innate signals. If you want that sticky bun, enjoy it, but have it once in a while – and no more. Just ensure that you eat it with the conscious knowledge that you're having sugar. Don't assume that your chiller-cabinet chicken or supermarket wholemeal bread is healthy – look on the pack and see what's in it.

STRATEGIES WHEN CRAVING

For those times when you do crave a sweet treat, try one of these alternatives:

Drink two large glasses of water
(some find sparkling water especially helpful)

Do some deep breathing
(such as 3–4–5 breathing, see page 50)

Distract yourself with a complex task that focuses
your attention elsewhere

Have a piece of fruit

Eat a handful of nuts

If you are really struggling, have a small portion of 90 per cent
(ideally 100 per cent) dark chocolate

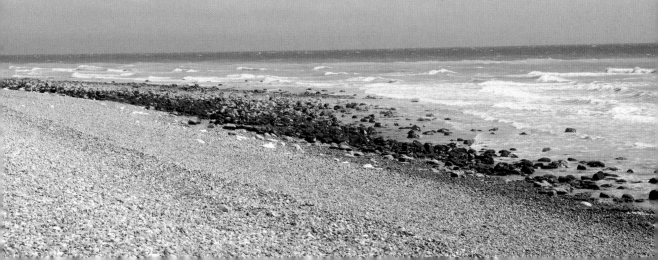

2. A NEW DEFINITION OF 'FIVE A DAY'

Aim to eat at least five portions of vegetables every day – ideally, of five different colours.

The UK government recommends eating five pieces of fruit and veg every single day. They allow fruit juice and smoothies as part of this, which I think is crazy. Given what we've just learned about sugar, and the fact that most juices are essentially liquid sugar, I believe this allowance is bizarre.

I prefer a different kind of five-a-day that involves eating five different types of vegetables. I'm always highly conscious of the scepticism many people feel when I pull this one out. They think this kind of intervention is somehow soft medicine. But, once again, it's based on hard science. It affects your body's biology in just the same way that a packet of pills you'd collect at the chemist's might.

My focus on vegetables alone doesn't mean I'm anti-fruit. I just find that, in an effort to get up their fruit and veg intake, most of my patients end up concentrating on super-sweet fruit. My food recommendations are intended partly to retune your palate. This approach will help you do that.

But why different vegetables of different colours? One of the reasons is that this variety is good for the bugs that live in our gut, and their associated genes, collectively known as our microbiome. Scientists have only recently begun focusing on this area, and it's becoming clear that the importance to our mental and physical health of having a healthy microbiome can hardly be overstated. And we have a lot of these bugs to feed. One 2014 paper found the human gut contains between

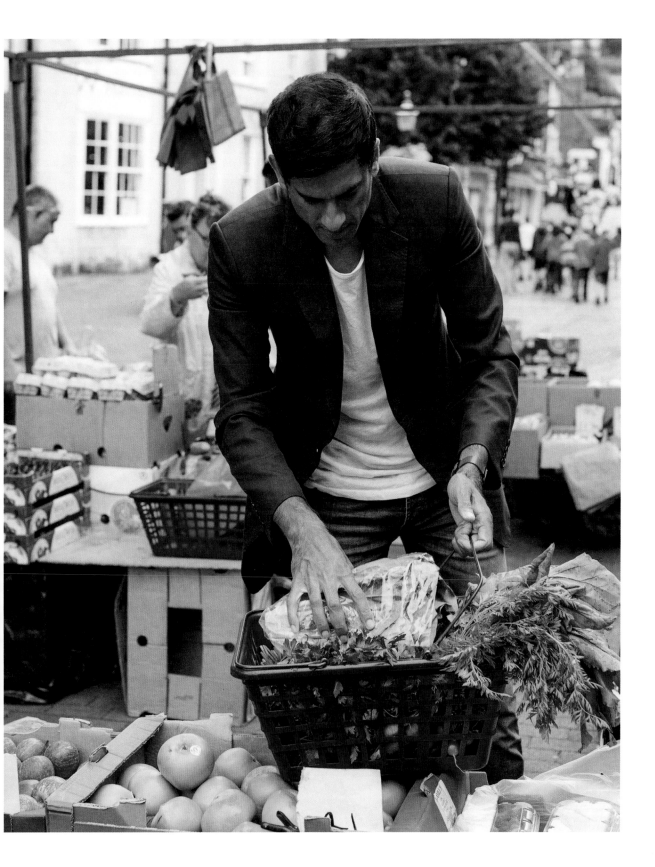

30 trillion and 400 trillion microorganisms whereas the number of actual human cells in our bodies ranges from 5 trillion to 724 trillion. 'Based upon these approximations,' write the scientists, 'the human body could have nearly the same amount of cells as microbes, or at the more extreme end, non-human cells may outnumber our own almost a hundred to one.' However, the really impressive numbers are found in the difference between the number of human genes we have compared with the number of microbial genes – in this case we are outnumbered by between a hundred and a thousand to one!

MICROBIOME DIVERSITY

The incredible complexity of our microbiome might mean that, in some cases, there are more 'non-human' cells in our bodies than actual human ones. Whilst researchers are discovering more about these bugs every day, there is still much that's unclear – not least what represents an ideal microbiome. Initially, the focus was on individual species of bugs to see which the 'good' bugs were and which the 'bad'. Eventually we realized this approach was almost certainly oversimplistic.

Our best guess at the moment is that an ideal microbiome is a diverse one, capable of adaptation and job share. These bugs have evolved with us over millions of years and live off the food we take in and, in return, provide a huge array of services to the human machine. For example, one species makes serotonin, which is the hormone linked with your mood. Others manufacture vitamins. Think of your own gut bug community as like staff in your factory that are producing the products you need to stay alive. That staff are made up of different specialists in different sections who are all expert in their own areas. To maintain optimal health, we need to ensure that all departments are adequately staffed. But we also need to make sure our teams are proportionate – that we have the right numbers of the right bugs and that no one team is over- or understaffed.

This is where we have a problem. Over the years our gut populations have been decimated by modern industrial living, food additives, high stress levels, the overuse of antibiotics and much more. We know this because studies have been carried out on populations that are still living largely as we once did. By peering inside their guts, we can get a decent idea of what our microbiomes may once have looked like. Studies on Amerindian populations suggest that those of us living in an industrialized society have lost at least a third of our gastrointestinal organisms. A recent examination of the Hadza, a Tanzanian hunter-gatherer tribe, suggested that the Western gut's microbiome is 50 per cent less diverse than theirs.

Whatever the figure, it seems clear we have much less diversity than we used to, and this is likely to be a key factor in our growing rates of chronic, degenerative disease. If we have a greatly diminished microbiome, it also might explain why we are no longer able to tolerate certain foods. This could also be a significant factor in the increasing amount of allergies and intolerances we're seeing. Currently, the UK scores in the top three countries in the world for the onset of allergies. Hay fever diagnoses have trebled over the last twenty years, whilst hospital admissions for allergies have increased by 500 per cent. It may not only be the food or the pollen that's the problem, but also the fact that the make-up of our microbiome has changed and with it, our capacity for environmental tolerance has declined.

To extend the metaphor, if a healthy microbiome has fully staffed departments all busily working on different functions, an unhealthy one has departments that have been shut down or are understaffed so not working effectively. Our microbiome represents a key component of our body's defence system against the outside world. The food we eat and its effect on our gut bugs is intimately linked with the activity of our body's immune system, all the more so, as the majority of our immune system is found in and around the gut. The fact that this critical component of our defence system has deteriorated at the same time that the quality of our food has reduced has, I believe, resulted in a perfect storm which may explain these rising numbers.

FEEDING YOUR MICROBIOME

There is a simple way we can start fixing our damaged microbiomes. We're forever being told that vegetables are good for us, but it's not often explained why. Well, here's one of the key reasons – because our gut bugs love plant-based fibre. This is also known as pre-biotic fibre. Broccoli is a particularly fine example. When the fibre that's in broccoli gets as far as your large bowel, or colon, it finds itself in the place where the vast majority of your gut bugs live. They feast on it and produce various by-products including short-chain fatty acids, or SCFAs. These SCFAs, including the most studied one, butyrate, are anti-inflammatory. This means that it helps bring down the inflammation whose harmful effects – including heart disease, stroke, Alzheimer's disease – we first heard about in the Relax pillar when discussing the importance of me-time and communal mealtimes. This is just a tiny part of that picture and it hopefully shows why simply thinking about diet in terms of calories, carbs and fat is so limiting.

BUILDING UP YOUR IMMUNE SYSTEM

Because the body is so interconnected, by feeding the microbiome we're also strengthening other parts of it, such as our immune system. It's common to think of the immune system as something that is there simply to protect us from airborne bacteria and viruses and prevent coughs and colds. Whilst that's true, 70 per cent of our immune system activity takes place in and around our gut. This makes perfect sense, of course, because our gut is one of the key interfaces between the external world and our bodies. According to one study, there are actually more immune reactions in your gut, over the course of one day, than in the rest of your body in your entire lifetime. This seems extraordinary until you remember that everything you put into your mouth is a foreign body.

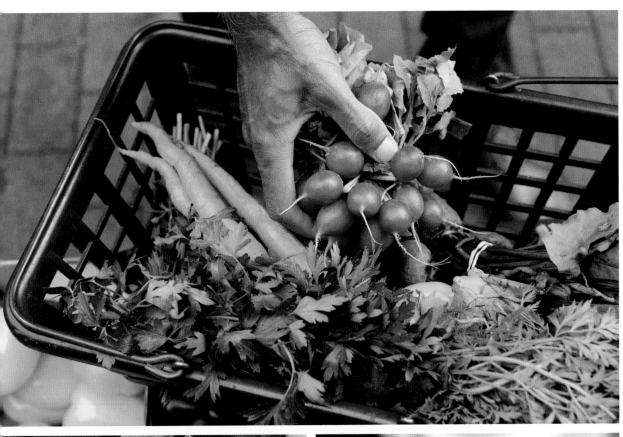

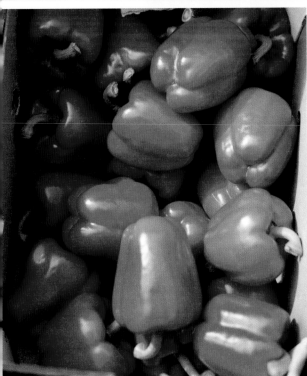

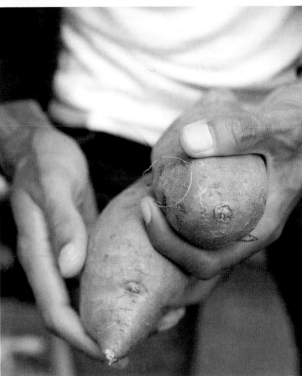

Specialized cells living in and around the gut lining use microscopic antennae to sample our food and check everything that passes through it. This information gathering, along with other signals, allows the immune system to make an active decision whether to let it in willingly or whether to react against it. If it reacts against it, the responses all involve the generation of inflammation and we can suffer myriad symptoms such as skin rashes, mood problems and joint pain. This happens because the system has become unruly and hypersensitive. You can think of the immune system as an army that's there to protect you from malevolent invaders. In a country that's in chaos, the army is out of control, overreacting and attacking everyone and everything – this is chronic inflammation. Eating certain foods can trigger the sending out of chemicals called cytokines that act as messengers, transmitting signals to the system that our bodies are under attack. But eating the right kind of foods can help bring that army back under control. It can give it order and discipline, making it more likely to attack only enemy targets and with a proportionate level of force.

Remember how good we said broccoli was as a means of feeding our microbiome? It also has a beneficial impact on our immune system. Before it even reaches the colon, where the gut bugs live, it arrives in the small intestine. On your small intestine you've got a kind of lock that will only take a particular key. This lock is called the aryl hydrocarbon receptor, or AHR. Certain vegetables – especially the cruciferous ones, such as cauliflower, broccoli, cabbage – have the correct key for the AHR lock. Bits of that broccoli will go into that AHR lock. When this happens, we get rewarded with a proliferation of what are called intraepithelial lymphocytes. These are fantastic, because they discipline your immune system. They calm it down, soothing the inflammation, helping ensure that it only responds when it needs to.

Our gut bugs and our immune system are not separate things operating in their own sectioned-off zones. They have a deep, powerful and historical interrelationship. There's even interplay between the composition of your gut bugs and the diet choices you make. That sounds incredible, I know, but your gut bugs can change your mood and these mood changes influence whether you're going to reach for the healthy salad or the super-sweet pastry. Eating different foods also affects your gut bugs in such a way that they alter our body's signalling processes, including how hungry you feel. In these ways and more, these trillions of bacteria that live inside you are taking over your thoughts and influencing your actions every day. It seems profoundly creepy, I know, but remember it works both ways. We can control our gut bugs – and help them work for us – with our food choices.

There are actually more immune reactions in your gut, over the course of one day, than the rest of your body in your entire lifetime.

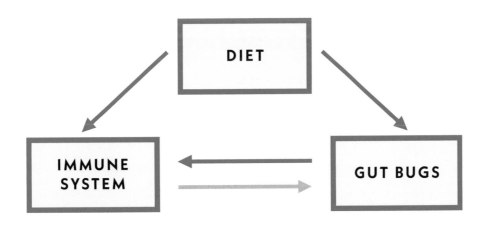

FOODS FOR YOUR GUT BUGS

Our ancestors ate between 50 and 150 grams of complex fibre per day – that is about 10 times the amount that most people eat today! These complex fibres are known as Microbiota Accessible Carbohydrates (MACs) because they are carbohydrates that feed our gut bugs. They're found in abundance in vegetables but also in fruits and legumes. We can't use them directly as they are hard to break down and digest. But our gut bugs can!

A recent study by experts from the University of Stanford found that because the modern Western diet is relatively low in MACs, we don't generate as many SCFAs as we should. As we've just discovered, these SCFAs are very important for many different healthy responses in the body, including reducing unwanted inflammation.

Every time you feel you can't eat any more veg – think about those little friends inside you. To feed yourself well, you need to feed your gut bugs well!

Although we still have a lot to learn about our gut bugs, there does appear to be one that almost certainly warrants the status of 'good' – Akkermansia muciniphila. Abundant studies show that the presence of this bug is associated with better weight control, insulin sensitivity and much more. Obese people tend to have less Akkermansia muciniphila than lean people. If we don't have enough of it we are at greater risk of becoming obese or diabetic. Remarkably, after weight loss surgery people's Akkermansia muciniphila levels increase. Whilst it's very hard to tease out cause and effect, it does appear that there is a compelling link between this particular gut bug and maintaining a healthy weight.

The gut has a protective lining of mucus that Akkermansia muciniphila feeds on, but it also feeds on:

- onions
- garlic
- leeks
- artichoke

- yams
- agave
- bananas
- Brussels sprouts

- okra
- cauliflower
- broccoli
- chicory root.

Akkermansia muciniphila adores these foods and will expand its numbers if fed accordingly. Fasting also leads to an increase in Akkermansia muciniphila, which is the subject of the next intervention.

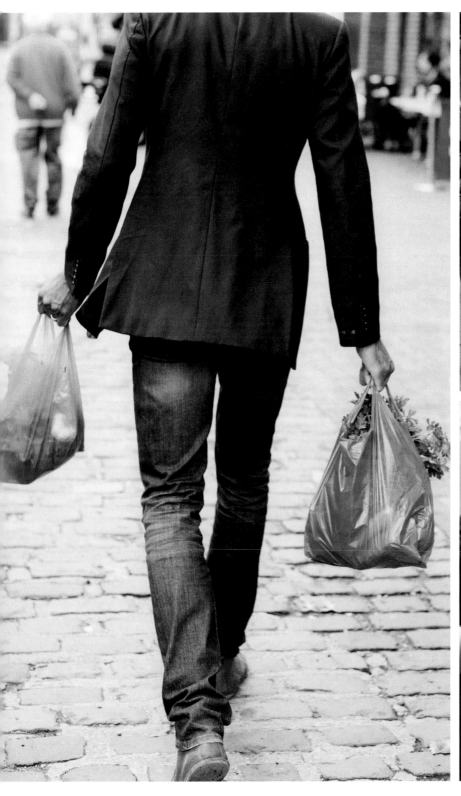
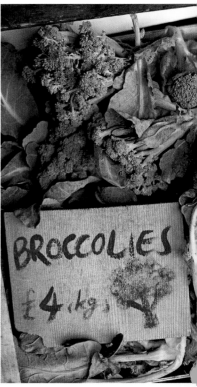
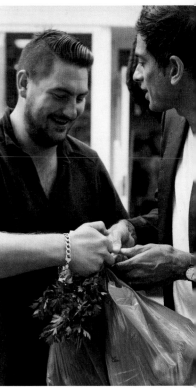

EATING THE RAINBOW

When you start eating differently, your microbiome will start changing within two to three days. Getting five different vegetables into your diet every single day will accelerate the process of optimizing your microbiome. To enhance the benefits even further, try to make these vegetables as many different colours as you can. This means it's much more likely that you will encourage the growth of more beneficial bacteria as well as getting maximum gut-bug diversity. But that's not the only benefit.

The more colours we eat, the more the variety we'll be getting of these incredible compounds that are known as phytonutrients. Many people don't like to eat their vegetables and vegetables themselves don't like to be eaten. Plants generate various compounds, called phytonutrients, to defend themselves against consumption. These defence molecules, when eaten by us, can have a remarkable impact on our health. There are literally thousands of them and we're only just beginning to understand their many benefits. They include many different types such as the polyphenols found in olives (see box on page 102) as well as the glucosinolates found in cruciferous vegetables such as broccoli, cauliflower, kale, turnips, Brussels sprouts and cabbage. We already know that phytonutrients help heart health, fight cancer cells, reduce inflammation and reverse brain ageing.

Different colours contain different phytonutrients. Red foods, such as tomatoes, contain lycopene, which some researchers argue reduces the risk of some types of cancer and heart disease. Orange foods, such as carrots, contain beta-carotene, which has a beneficial effect on our immune system and promotes healthy vision. Green vegetables, such as broccoli, contain chlorophyll, which seems to help control hunger. The phytonutrients found in bitter foods such as kale help us feel full. The list goes on. (You even find polyphenols – a particular type of phytonutrient – in delightful products like red wine, coffee and high-quality chocolate – but that's not an excuse to binge!)

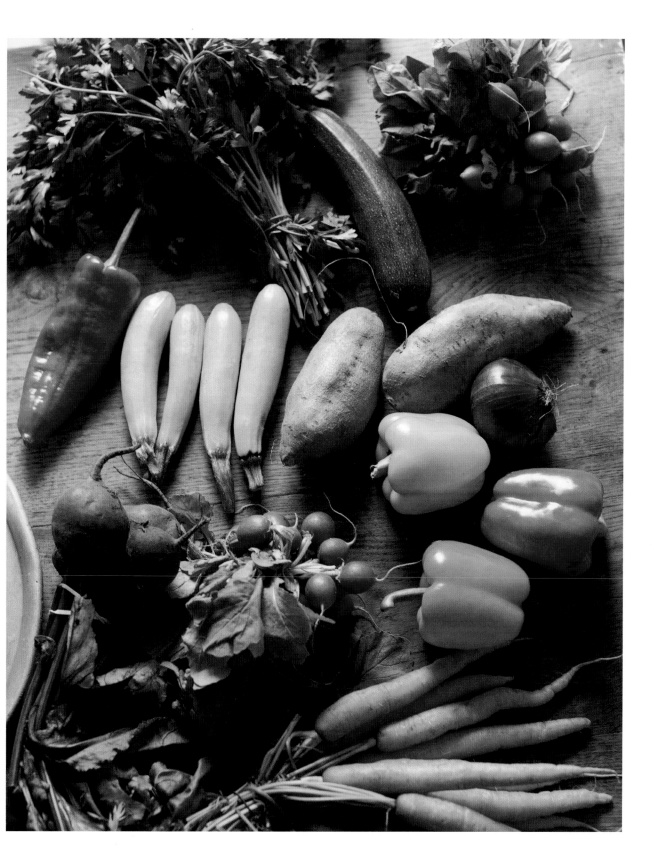

POLYPHENOLS

Polyphenols are a special class of phytonutrients. There are many different types of polyphenol including lignans from flax seeds, flavonoids found in dark chocolate and red wine, catechins found in tea, and anthocyanins found in broccoli and berries. We're only just beginning to learn about the many different health benefits they confer.

So far we do know that polyphenols have powerful antioxidant effects. Oxidation is a normal process that occurs in the body as a by-product of various physiological functions. If the antioxidant balance is disrupted the result in our bodies can very simplistically be likened to rusting on a car. Polyphenols help to dampen down this rusting process and prevent it causing damage to our bodies.

Other health benefits may include:

Lower inflammation	Improved blood sugar control
Slower ageing	Improved cardiovascular health
Reduced blood pressure	Healthier microbiome
Improved brain health	Improved immune function

Vegetables
One of the best ways to increase the amount of polyphenols in your diet is by eating brightly coloured fibre-rich vegetables. The best sources are spinach, broccoli, red onions, asparagus, red lettuce, shallots, carrots, artichokes and both green and black olives. Polyphenols are typically found in higher concentrations in the skin of fruit and vegetables, so peeling them can remove a large amount.

Berries

Berries are worth a special mention as they are jam-packed full of polyphenols. I actually highly recommend berries to my patients because of their high polyphenol content in addition to their five vegetables per day. Their bright colours also make it easier for you to eat the rainbow.

Other sources

Some of the best sources include dark chocolate, coffee and nuts such as pecans and hazelnuts. The polyphenols found in black and green tea can inhibit the growth of many problematic gut bugs. You can also up your intake with the liberal use of herbs, especially rosemary, thyme and peppermint, and by using copious amounts of extra virgin olive oil.

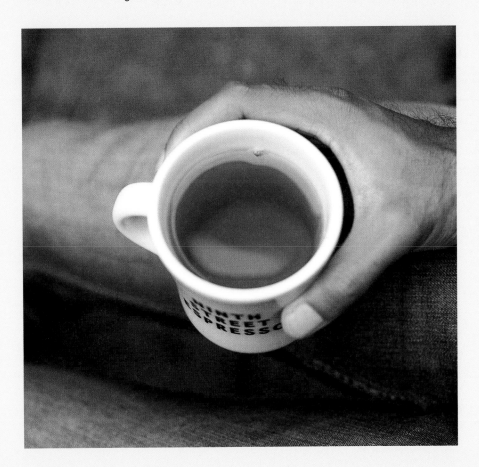

HOW TO INCREASE YOUR COLOURS

Use the rainbow chart on pages 106–7 to help increase the number of colours you consume. My focus with this intervention is primarily to encourage you to eat five different vegetables per day. If you can make them different colours too, so much the better. I have included some non-vegetable items in the chart such as blueberries, nuts, lentils and black rice because of their established health benefits. My hope is that these additional items will help to make your diet more colourful.

Here are some practical tips to help increase your vegetable intake and variety:

- Print out the rainbow chart from drchatterjee.com and put it on your fridge. Tick off all the colours you have consumed in one day.

- Involve friends, family or work colleagues to help you stay motivated.

- Get in the habit of snacking on veg – carrots with hummus, cucumber with tahini, celery sticks with almond butter are some tasty options.

- Avocados and olives make a quick and easy snack – although technically fruits, in culinary circles they are treated as vegetables. I consider them to be foods that can be included as part of your new 'five a day'.

- Leave colourful, appealing vegetables on the kitchen worktop or your desk so that you see them regularly: bright orange carrots, slices of red and yellow peppers, green olives.

- Add two vegetables to every meal, including breakfast. If you're having eggs in the morning, try adding spinach and avocado.

- A tip that I use with my children is to serve them their vegetables first. Only when they have eaten them will I dish out the rest of the meal. This works for adults too!

- Roast a whole baking tray of colourful vegetables drizzled with olive oil; eat some with your evening meal and save leftovers in the fridge. They can form the basis of lunch the next day.

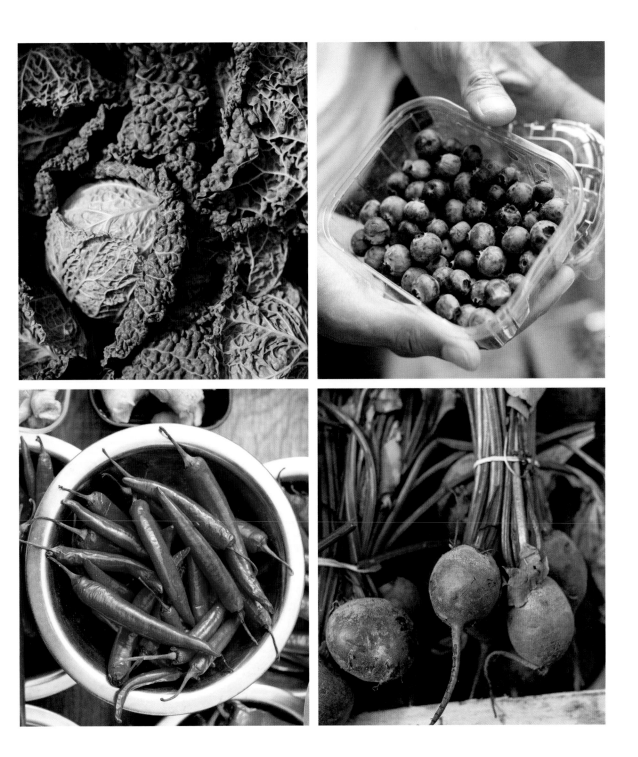

RAINBOW CHART FOR YOU TO COMPLETE

ARTICHOKE	CUCUMBER	RED PEPPERS
ASPARAGUS	EDAMAME BEANS	BEETROOT
AVOCADO	GREEN BEANS	RED ONIONS
BAMBOO SHOOTS	GARDEN PEAS	RED CABBAGE
GREEN PEPPERS	ROCKET	RADISH
BOK CHOY	SPINACH	RHUBARB
BROCCOLI	LETTUCE	TOMATO
BRUSSELS SPROUTS	SWISS CHARD	RADICCHIO
CABBAGE	KALE	
CELERY	OKRA	

MONDAY

TUESDAY

WEDNESDAY

THURSDAY

FRIDAY

SATURDAY

SUNDAY

CARROTS		OLIVES	CHICKPEAS
ORANGE PEPPERS	SWEETCORN	PURPLE CARROTS	CAULIFLOWER
PUMPKIN	YELLOW PEPPERS	PURPLE SWEET POTATOES	MUSHROOMS
BUTTERNUT SQUASH	GINGER ROOT	KALE	SHALLOTS
SWEET POTATO	SUMMER SQUASH	PURPLE POTATOES	SEEDS
TURMERIC ROOT	LEMONS	BLUEBERRIES	ONIONS
		RED CABBAGE	GARLIC
		BLACK RICE	TURNIPS
		AUBERGINE	FENNEL
			NUTS
			LENTILS
			PARSNIPS

3. INTRODUCE DAILY MICRO-FASTS

Get into the habit of eating all of your food within a twelve-hour time window.

Humans evolved during periods of regular feast and famine. Our bodies are designed for going without food for certain periods of time. But the modern environment, in which we're surrounded by temptations to eat – be they social pressures, via advertising or the simple fact we have that delicious half-eaten trifle sitting in our fridge – means we tend to inundate our systems.

As soon as you start to give your body a break from all the gorging, incredible things start to happen. An extraordinary health-promoting cascade effect is triggered. After six to eight hours, the liver will have used up its internal fuel stores, in the form of glycogen, and soon after this the body will start to burn its own fat. Once we get to about twelve hours, a process called autophagy will have well and truly kicked in.

Autophagy is another hot area of new research that I wasn't taught about at medical school. Much of what we know about it is thanks to the Japanese biologist Yoshinori Ohsumi, who won the Nobel Prize for Medicine for his work into its mechanisms. Imagine that you never spent time cleaning up your house. You'd leave dirty plates hanging around for weeks, stinky clothes on the floor, kids' toys everywhere, washing baskets overflowing, the sinks machine-gunned with toothpaste splats. This is basically what happens in the body, every day, as a by-product of it going about its daily functions. The scientific term for this is 'oxidative damage'. It's actually a little bit like the rust that builds up on cars. This build-up is an inevitable consequence of function – and it's all fine as long as we give our body a chance to clean up. This is what autophagy does. Think of it as your built-in Cinderella. It's your body sorting out its mess and busying itself with cellular repair, immune system repair and a host of other essential maintenance projects. Eating all your food in a restricted time window – for example, within twelve hours – allows your body to enhance its own natural house-cleaning.

Being such a new area of science, there's still limited data on human studies into exactly how and why time-restricted feeding (TRF) assists our repair processes. However, one likely mechanism that's been proposed is that when we don't eat for several hours, the liver stops secreting glucose into the bloodstream and instead uses it to repair cell damage. The liver is simultaneously stimulated to release enzymes that break down stored fat and cholesterol. Therefore, during our fasting period, the liver is helping to repair our bodies and burn off fat!

And these are by no means the only benefits of restricting our hours of eating. An incredible American neurologist, Professor Dale Bredesen, has actually managed to reverse memory loss in early-Alzheimer's patients by taking a multipronged approach that has, as an essential component, regular twelve-hour fasts. Yet more compelling research is coming out of the lab of Dr Satchidananda Panda, a biologist at the Salk Institute for Biological Studies in San Diego. Dr Panda is a passionate promoter of the idea that restricting the timing of our food intake may be an extremely effective public health stratagem. He argues that simply trying to eliminate unhealthy foods and restrict calories hasn't really proved successful – so perhaps a limited eating window might work better.

If all that wasn't enough, early studies are showing that when animals are given exactly the same diets over varying time periods, the metabolic effects on their body are significantly different – they put on less fat and have larger muscle mass when they are fed over a shorter period. This is hugely exciting. Human trials are under way.

So far the reported benefits are:

Lower levels of inflammation

Improved blood sugar control

Improved mitochondrial function (see box opposite)

Improved immune function

Enhanced detoxification – TRF improves the elimination of waste products

Increased production of Akkermansia muciniphila (see page 98)

Improved appetite signalling

It is possible to enhance these benefits by shortening our eating window even further, but I recommend twelve hours because fasting for longer can be problematic for some. Most patients I see are chronically overstressed. They need more rest-and-recuperation time, not more time under stress. Although perhaps not truly optimal, twelve hours is both manageable and long enough for most of us to see real benefits.

Which twelve hours should you choose? Recently I experimented by not eating after 7 p.m. I found it surprisingly easy. As it turned out, eating later was just habit, just as feeling hungry later was a habit, mostly based upon the readily available access to food in my house. When I stopped eating during the evenings I felt more energetic, had better sleep and was just generally a little lighter in myself. I came to think of that evening craving for food as having a kind of 'itchy mouth'. That's become the way we talk about it in my house now. Am I really hungry? Or do I just have an itchy mouth?

MITOCHONDRIA

Mitochondria are the energy factories of your body. Every cell contains hundreds of thousands of them. They convert fuel, in the form of oxygen and food, into energy. If we want to reach optimal health, we should try to enhance mitochondrial function in any way we can.

Most mitochondria are found in highly active organs such as the brain and the heart and in muscle tissue. Mitochondrial function is central to almost every single physiological process in the body.

Poor mitochondrial function can result in:

- Low energy level
- Brain fog
- Pain
- Poor memory
- Premature ageing

As mitochondria produce energy, reactive oxygen species (ROS) are formed. These cause oxidation, which is a bit like rusting on a car. In order to mop these potentially harmful reactive oxygen species up, our bodies need to produce sufficient antioxidants from the fruit and vegetables in our diet. Small amounts of these ROS are helpful, but too many causes problems.

When mitochondria don't function optimally, the increase in ROS is known as increased oxidative stress.

In the short or medium term, this can contribute to the symptoms listed above such as fatigue and poor memory. Over the long term, this leads to chronic inflammation which can be a significant driver of many different diseases in the body including obesity, type 2 diabetes and stroke.

Eating an anti-inflammatory wholefood diet (see 'Unprocess your diet' on page 124) helps provide mitochondria with the correct fuel and necessary repair materials. In addition, the mitochondrial walls are made up of fat, so having healthy sources of natural fat in your diet such as avocados, olive oil and oily fish is important. They also need the right fuel, which can be obtained from eating an anti-inflammatory wholefood diet.

WORKING WITH YOUR CIRCADIAN RHYTHM

Although the science in this area is still in its infancy, human studies are already hinting that scheduling an earlier evening meal, or skipping it completely, may be more beneficial than not having breakfast. This appears to be because certain bodily functions shut down and don't function optimally in the evening. Intuitively, this makes a lot of sense, but in the scientific world this is actually quite surprising. Isn't a body like a machine? As in, it either works or it doesn't? Why should one bit of it work better at a certain time of day?

I find it incredibly exciting that much of our biological machinery actually has its own daily cycle, not dissimilar to the one that makes us feel sleepy or alert at different points of the day. Even if we're not deeply familiar with the science of the 'circadian rhythm' – how the body floods with melatonin to make us drowsy and cortisol to wake us up – we'll certainly be aware of its effects. It's now becoming clear that our bodies work on any number of these kinds of routine cycles.

Last year I was on my way to a conference in San Diego and, on the plane from Manchester to Heathrow, I happened to find myself sitting next to Andrew Louden, a professor of animal biology from the University of Manchester. We started chatting and before I knew it, we'd landed. We both had some time to wait before our next flight so continued the conversation over coffee. As I sipped at my short black Americano, I mentioned I was travelling to a conference on sleep-cycles and I started talking to him about body clocks. 'Well, yes, I actually study body clocks,' he chuckled. 'And it's not all about sleep, you know. Did you know that if you take a bunch of human liver cells and put them in a test tube, they start operating by daily rhythms?'

I found this extraordinary. Andrew told me that all of our bodily functions are determined by a circadian rhythm. This made me wonder if one potentially major failing of many health and nutrition studies might be that they haven't accounted for this. When I looked into it, I found some fascinating recent research to suggest that certain pharmaceutical drugs could work better at different times of the day. Certain genes are also more or less active at various points. Even the composition of our gut microbiome changes with the hours. Interestingly enough, traditional Chinese medicine has been making this kind of observation for thousands of years. They've long believed that various organs have increased function at certain times of the day.

All this explains why it's a good idea to start your time-restricted feeding window earlier. Hunter-gatherers tended to do their 'work' either in the morning or at twilight. Have our bodies kept this ancient programming and could this be one of the reasons that gene activity, for example, peaks at these times? I don't think we know the exact answer to this question yet, but it seems logical. If you ask me, we're not meant to be eating just before we're about to go to bed. We've evolved to eat in the light. Indeed, researchers in Scandinavia found that, in some people, when the body is preparing to sleep, and we're feeling tired, the pancreas stops making insulin. You can't override that. Today, we're eating out of sync with our natural rhythms. Time-restricted feeding helps us readjust and give the body what it's expecting at the time it's expecting it. This helps it make the most efficient use of the fuel we swallow.

SIX TIPS TO HELP YOU MICRO-FAST

1. Choose a twelve-hour period that suits your lifestyle. Note that your twelve-hour eating window is from the beginning of your first meal to the end of your last meal.

2. Your body likes rhythm, so try and keep to the same times every day, even at weekends. Occasionally you may need to change your eating window – this is absolutely fine.

3. Outside your eating window, stick to water, herbal tea or black tea and coffee. Be careful with caffeine so you don't adversely affect your sleep (see page 244).

4. Try to involve other members of your household, or even work colleagues. This will help to keep you motivated and increase your chances of success.

5. Don't be disheartened if you miss a day, or even two. It really doesn't matter. When you feel ready, try again and see how you get on.

6. When you are feeling comfortable with twelve hours, you may choose to experiment with shorter eating windows on different days. If you do this, pay attention to how the change makes you feel and adjust accordingly.

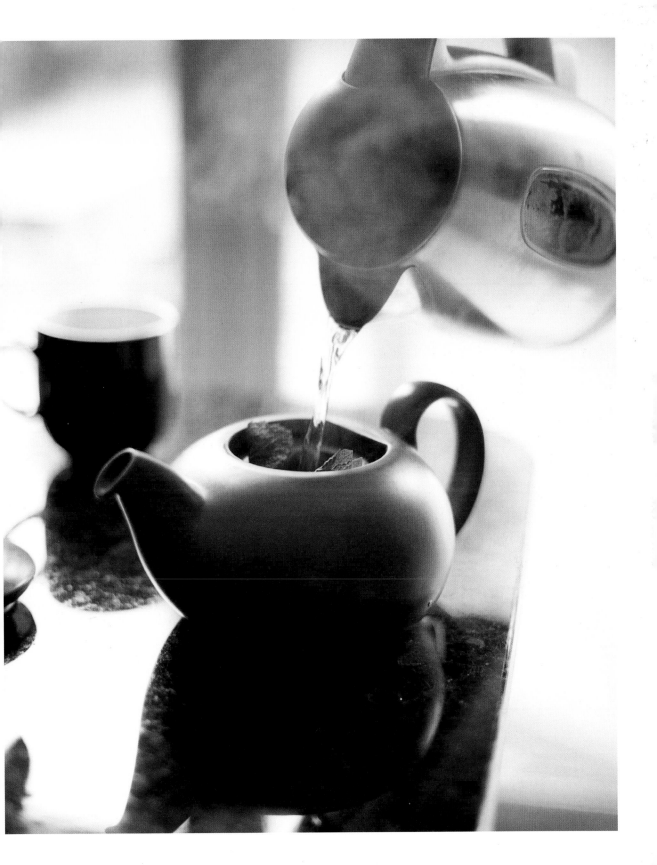

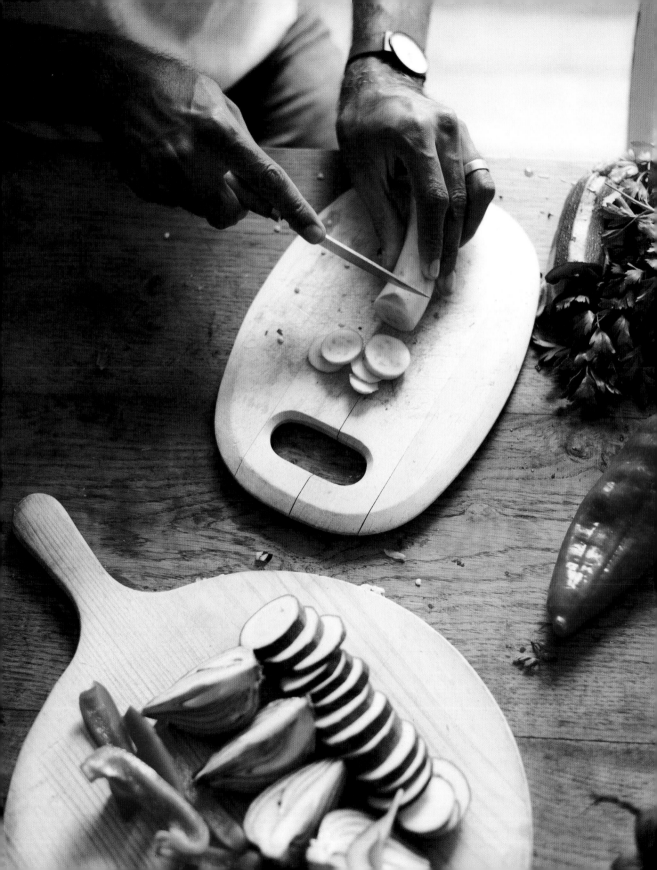

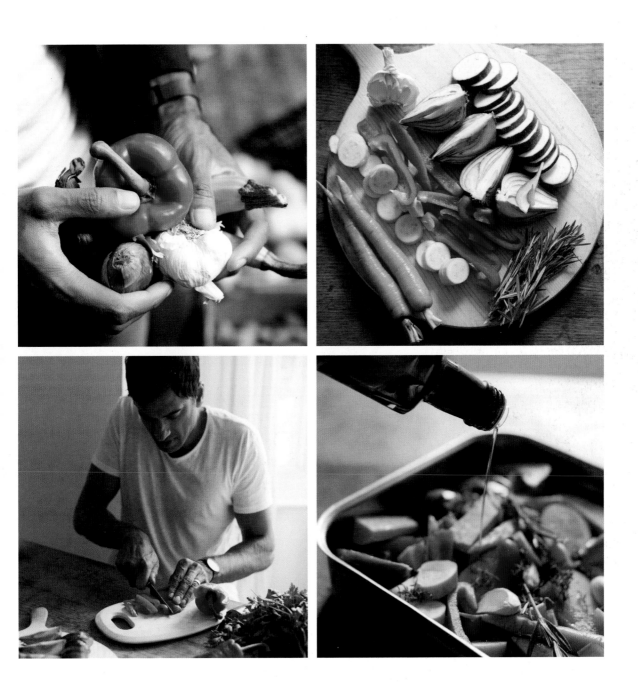

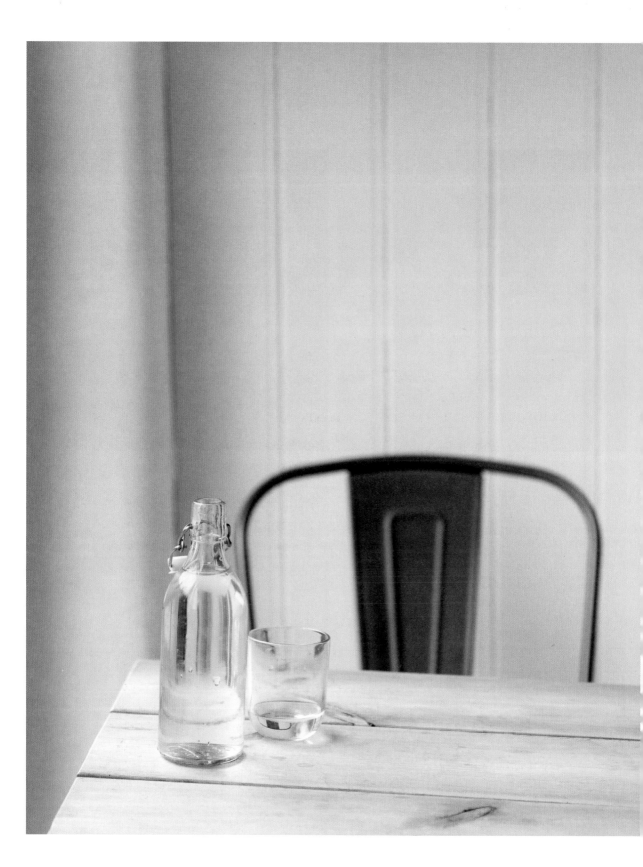

4. DRINK MORE WATER

Aim to drink eight small glasses (approximately 1.2 litres)
of water per day.

Do you feel tired? Or regularly experience low-grade and long-lasting headaches? Often when worried patients come in complaining of symptoms such as these, it turns out that many of them are simply not drinking enough water.

Now the idea we should be drinking eight glasses of water a day has been around for many years but, interestingly enough, there's not actually that much science to support it. That doesn't mean I'm not going to recommend it, however. What should I do as a practising doctor? Wait for the evidence to come from academia that frankly may never arrive? Or should I make a sensible recommendation that I've seen help thousands of patients? I choose to help patients now.

This is the big difference between researchers and clinicians. Researchers assess evidence but it can be a long time before such evidence gets translated into mainstream clinical practice – some say about thirty years! In addition, some concepts never get properly examined, sometimes because they're hard to study, but often because there's simply no financial imperative to do so. I always remember my chat with the inspiring Olympic strength coach Charles Poliquin: 'If you wait for the evidence, you may miss three Olympic cycles,' he told me. That idea has resonated with me ever since.

HOW MUCH WATER SHOULD WE BE DRINKING?

In America, they've been recommending eight eight-ounce glasses of water every day for a number of years. This equates to about 1.9 litres. This does appear to be quite a lot and I'm not necessarily sure we all need to be chugging down as much as that. In the UK, though, our glasses are a bit smaller. When we have eight glasses we're looking at about 1.2 litres of water, which is probably much closer to a practical ideal.

About 60 per cent of the body is made up of water and we can only last a few days without it. Water helps us digest food and process substances such as alcohol. Losing just 2 per cent of body weight in fluid can actually reduce our physical and mental performance by up to 25 per cent. I've seen a host of different ailments clear up when people start drinking more water, including headaches, low energy levels, dry skin and tummy ache. It can even be helpful for constipation. If you're feeling tired and sluggish in the afternoon, it could simply be that you are slightly dehydrated. I've experienced this myself on many occasions (at least whilst writing this book).

DON'T DRINK YOUR CALORIES

As someone who abides by the Hippocratic oath, one of my first criteria with any recommendation I make is, how much harm can it do? The only potential downside to this one is maybe a couple more trips to the toilet. But that's it, and even that helps you increase your daily activity level, which I'd chalk up as a benefit. In addition, drinking more water will hopefully mean you start drinking less of the sweetened stuff, such as juices and soft drinks. Fluid bypasses normal satiety mechanisms in the body and allows us to consume a lot more energy and calories than would be possible if we were eating. Think about oranges as an example. A glass of orange juice could easily have six or seven oranges in it. It's perfectly possible to drink a whole glass in one go whereas it's very difficult to eat six or seven oranges at a sitting. Whole oranges also contain fibre that slows the release of sugar into the body. Juicing removes that beneficial fibre.

And don't think you can necessarily get around this by sticking to diet drinks. A correlation has been found between zero-calorie soft drinks and disorders such as diabetes. Whilst the science isn't able to say definitively that drinking these products causes these problems, it certainly remains a distinct possibility. There are several plausible mechanisms we know of that could explain how this might happen. One theory has it that diet drinks contain chemicals that can have an adverse impact on the gut microbiome. As we've already learned, our microbiome health is critical for good health. Whilst we're waiting for the science catch-up, I'd advocate not taking the risk, and cutting out diet drinks too.

A patient of mine named Annabelle had been suffering from headaches for years and had tried many different medications unsuccessfully. These headaches didn't really follow any pattern and she was getting extremely frustrated by them. When I first met her, I got the sense that she wasn't drinking enough water. I asked her to aim for eight glasses per day. In less than a week, her headaches completely vanished. An added bonus was that she had more energy as well.

Again, I must stress that I'm aware of no study that points to eight glasses as being optimal. It's simply impossible for me to state with accuracy what your individual requirements are. It depends on so many variables, including the kind of job you have, the physical size of your body and even the climate in which you live. But in my years of clinical experience I've found that eight glasses seems to be about right for most people, most of the time. A simple rule of thumb is to look at your urine. You're aiming for a colour that is light yellow to clear.

Many people – my father-in-law included – find it extremely difficult to get anywhere near eight glasses of water per day. For people like him, I've come up with some simple strategies. First thing in the morning drink two glasses. If you'd prefer some flavour in it, try squeezing some lemon in there. Before you've even started filling up with breakfast, you're already two glasses down. Another helpful strategy is to add in a glass of water thirty minutes before each meal. There is some evidence suggesting that drinking water thirty minutes before meals may reduce the amount of calories you consume. Then, if you start feeling hunger pangs in the middle of the morning or mid-afternoon, try having a couple of glasses of water instead between meals.

If you implement some of the above strategies, you should be well on your way in no time.

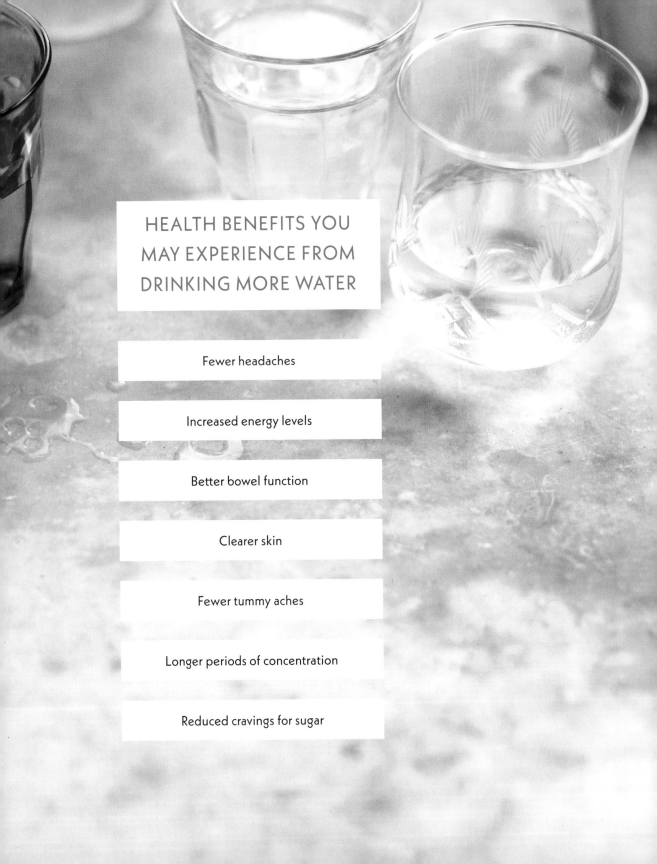

HEALTH BENEFITS YOU MAY EXPERIENCE FROM DRINKING MORE WATER

Fewer headaches

Increased energy levels

Better bowel function

Clearer skin

Fewer tummy aches

Longer periods of concentration

Reduced cravings for sugar

TIPS TO HELP YOU INCREASE
YOUR WATER INTAKE

HAVE TWO GLASSES OF WATER WHEN YOU WAKE UP
EACH MORNING

IF YOU'RE HUNGRY MID-MORNING OR MID-AFTERNOON, TRY HAVING
A GLASS OF WATER INSTEAD OF A SNACK

ONCE EVERY HOUR, GET UP FROM YOUR DESK AND GO TO THE
WATER COOLER

DRINK A GLASS OF WATER THIRTY MINUTES BEFORE EACH MEAL

SET AN ALARM THREE TIMES PER DAY TO REMIND YOU
TO HAVE A DRINK

TRY ADDING LEMON OR ORANGE SLICES FOR FLAVOUR

BUY A 600ML WATER BOTTLE. WE'RE AIMING FOR 1.2 LITRES
PER DAY, SO TRY TO HAVE FINISHED ONE BY LUNCH AND
ONE BY TEATIME

5. UNPROCESS YOUR DIET

Try to avoid food products that contain more than five ingredients.

There's no need to count calories, portion size, fats, carbs, Weight Watchers points, Slimmer's World 'sins' or anything even remotely like that. Life is complicated enough as it is. Instead, simply focus on avoiding highly processed foods. It's a pretty safe bet that any food product that contains more than five ingredients is highly processed. By avoiding these foods you will, by default, be not only improving your health but also side-stepping all the endless confusion that exists about diet. All you need to do is remember the number five.

Our ideas about food have become too reductionist. We've been beguiled by powerful diet cults that are desperate to convert us to their passionate belief that they have found the One True Diet. Everyone – including me – has been swept up in these debates and harbours their own personal biases about what's good and bad. For years we were told that the answer lay in counting calories, despite the fact that a healthy avocado contains more than double the calories of a can of Coke. Do they both have the same effect on the body? Of course not. (And we know which has more than five ingredients!)

We've also been led to believe that all our dietary problems can be solved by controlling one single component of them, be it fat or carbs. I believe that the major problem is not that we're simply eating too much food; it's actually that we're eating the wrong type of food. Our culinary environment has changed to the point that we are now eating large quantities of low-quality food. I'm convinced that by simply focusing on quality, many of our problems, including obesity and diabetes, will simply fall away.

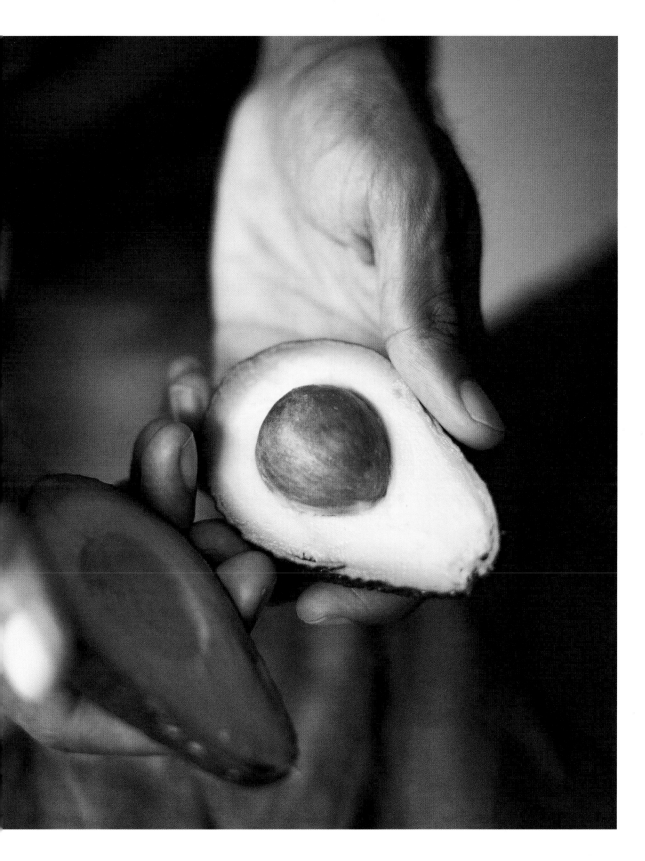

LOW-CARB DIETS

I know that many of you will now be thinking, 'Well I've lost plenty of weight and become healthier on a low-carb diet.' I don't doubt it. Today, of course, there's a burgeoning low-carb movement that's spread across much of the world. By and large, I support many aspects of this movement but I tend not to use the phrase 'low carb'. I think that we've unfairly demonized fat for nearly fifty years and I'm worried that we're now making the same mistake with carbs. I also think some of its more inflexible proponents focus too much on how many carbs we eat. For me, it's not about simply the quantity of carbs in our diet. It's about the quality.

The reality is that the majority of carbs we're now exposed to in the West, such as bread, pasta, muffins, cakes and biscuits, are refined and ultra-processed. They have become a daily staple – you can't even buy a cup of coffee these days without having to run the gauntlet of tempting treats. The problem is not necessarily that they are carbs, it's that they're poor quality carbs. In the blue zone of Okinawa, Japan, for example, people eat a diet high in healthy carbs and are known for their longevity. The case of the Okinawans is clear and powerful evidence that demonizing carbs in and of themselves is simplistic and misguided.

LOW-FAT DIETS

Supporters of the low-carb movement tend to be critics of the low-fat movement. They argue that low fat didn't work because people replaced fat with carbs. Yet there are many who swear that their health improves when consuming a low-fat diet. Many proponents of this tend to favour foods that are 'plant-based' and low in animal products, if not entirely free from them, such as with vegan diets. I've seen many patients transition from a highly processed Western diet to a low-fat, plant-based diet and do very well.

So who's right? Are you confused? Don't be. The bottom line is that if you increase the amount of low-quality foods in your diet, be it fat, carbs, or protein, your health will inevitably suffer. Just remember that highly processed foods – including most of those with more than five ingredients – can be extremely damaging to us, and can cause any number of health problems via a chain reaction, which will ultimately affect every process in your body.

(Note: this intervention is about encouraging you to eat more unprocessed wholefoods. You are free, and actively encouraged, to cook a meal yourself that contains more than five ingredients. The key is to avoid food *products* that contain more than five.)

A UNIQUE ROLE FOR LOW-CARB DIETS

When comparing the diets of populations around the world, we often miss out other important factors that play a critical role in health – physical activity levels, sleep quality, stress levels and how much vitamin D they might be getting from being out in the sun every day. These factors all play an important role in determining not only how healthy you are but also the kind of diet you need to thrive.

The Okinawans who do so well on a high-carb diet also get a lot of sunshine and sleep, engage in physical activity and have a strong sense of community as well as low levels of stress. As you know by now, good health results from not just a single component but a combination of many factors that will enable you to reach your own personal threshold.

Could it be that in the modern Western world, where so many of us are deficient in sunlight (which gives us vitamin D as well as much more), too sedentary, sleep deprived, overstressed and, on top of all that, constantly shovelling large amounts of processed carbohydrates down our throats, a low-carb diet serves a particular and unique role?

Perhaps it is in this environment where they have their greatest effect. Maybe in Okinawa, they can reach their threshold another way?

LEAKY GUT

A state of increased intestinal permeability, colloquially known as 'leaky gut', is something that I am seeing more and more of in my surgery. To start this story, I first need to explain some key functions of the digestive system. When you consume food, it travels down an elongated tube called the digestive tract. This tract is separated from our bloodstream by a border. This border is extremely thin but also extremely well protected. It's made up of tightly packed cells called mucosal cells.

When these mucosal cells are stuck together correctly, they form a protective barrier between the outside world and our bloodstream. To actually get through this barrier requires our food to become fully digested into very small particles. Only then does it pass through these tightly packed cells and enter our bloodstream. But there's another line of protection waiting for it there. On the other side of this border sits the immune system. One of the immune system's roles is to test our food and react accordingly.

If you're eating the right kinds of foods, this system will be working well and you'll probably have an excellent level of protection. When you're eating poor-quality food, the tightly packed mucosal cells that make up your border can become loose and your gut becomes leaky. This means that morsels of food can slip between or through the mucosal cells that make up our barrier and adversely trigger the immune system which becomes overwhelmed. This makes you vulnerable to ill-health.

Imagine going through security at an airport. If you walk through the sensor without triggering it, you pick up your stuff on the other side and safely go on your way. But if there's something in your hand luggage that the security system is suspicious of, an alarm will sound. You'll have to wait in line whilst someone rummages through your luggage. It'll likely be stressful and frustrating. Your cortisol will rise. Your heart will pound. You might even miss your flight. Ultimately, you'll be let through, but at a cost. This is a bit like the process that's triggered when we eat highly processed food. Alarm signals are triggered in the body. The muffins or burgers get digested, but there's a price to pay.

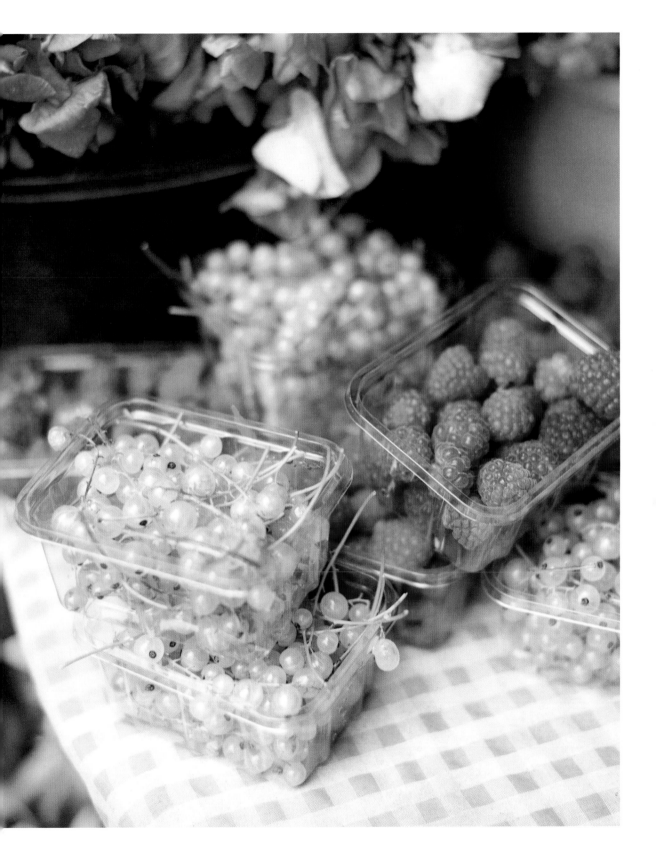

LPS THE MENACE

Leaky gut can lead to all kinds of other problems, including bloating and heartburn, as well as problems further afield, such as joint pain, skin complaints such as eczema, obesity and even depression. What's more, if you have a leaky gut, some particularly nasty molecules called lipopolysaccharides, or LPSs, can slip into your system. LPSs are found naturally on the walls of certain kinds of gut bacteria but they're not supposed to be in our blood. They're actually highly toxic. If you inject LPSs into someone's veins their blood pressure will plummet and they'll go into a coma.

If LPSs slip through your gut barrier the effects are not quite as dramatic. However, the longer-term impacts can be just as serious. LPSs alarm your immune system, which then sends out inflammatory cytokines throughout the body. This puts your body's inbuilt security systems on high alert. This consumes vital energy resources and increases your risk of poor health.

This ongoing, unresolved inflammation is problematic. In our airport, the sirens would be blaring loudly, everyone would be getting stopped and searched and flights would be leaving empty or being cancelled. There would be chaos. In its efforts to protect you, the whole system can run out of control. This helps to explain why the presence of LPSs in our blood has been associated with a wide variety of health problems ranging from joint pain and obesity to type 2 diabetes, as well as autoimmune conditions such as rheumatoid arthritis and neurodegenerative conditions such as Alzheimer's. Many of these share chronic inflammation as a common driver.

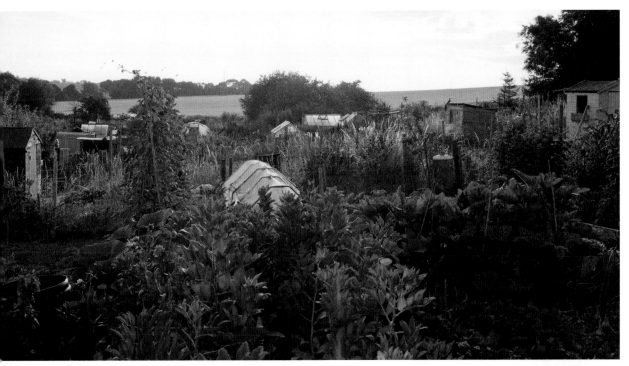

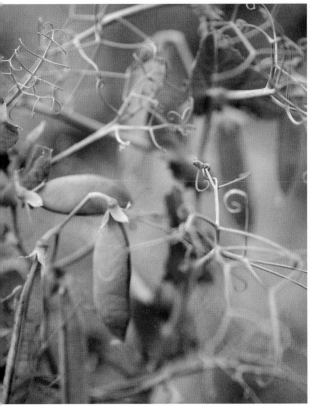

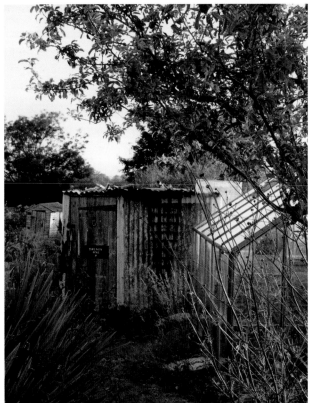

INFLAMMATION

Inflammation is one of the fundamental ways in which we defend and repair ourselves.

If you sprain your ankle, it gets hot, swollen and red. This is acute inflammation and helps the area heal. A short while after, when the body has completed its healing, the inflammation is switched off. So far, so good.

Inflammation is meant to be a short-lived process that protects us. It becomes problematic when it's longstanding and unresolved. That is what's happening to many of us as a result of our modern lives – our bodies believe they are constantly under attack. Our lifestyles are sending the body stress signals that trigger the body's defence systems.

This is one of the major reasons why our society is so sick. Chronic inflammation is behind the development of many modern, degenerative diseases.

A brilliant 2013 paper from Australia looked at the link between chronic inflammation and depression. Its authors reviewed a wealth of data that explored how lifestyle problems such as stress, lack of sleep, physical inactivity and poor diet as well as gut permeability and smoking can drive inflammation which, in turn, can increase the risk of depression. They concluded, 'Most of these factors are plastic, and potentially amenable to therapeutic and preventative interventions.' In other words, by making the lifestyle interventions I recommend to bring inflammation back down, it looks like, in many cases, we can actually treat depression and other inflammation-driven illnesses.

The basic principles are identical to those outlined in *The Four Pillar Plan*:

* Reduce processed food and eat an anti-inflammatory diet (see opposite)

* Eat more plant-based fibre to support a healthy and diverse microbiome

* Prioritize regular and consistent sleep

* Reduce and manage stress, both physical and emotional

* Increase your physical activity

THE ANTI-INFLAMMATORY DIET

The science of inflammation and gut permeability has led me to what I believe is a major new perspective on health and nutrition. I'm convinced the idea of the anti-inflammatory diet is potentially revolutionary. As we know, chronic, ongoing inflammation is a key driver of the epidemic of lifestyle-driven diseases that we're currently in the midst of. I think that damaged fats (such as vegetable oils, which can degrade when heated) as well as the highly refined carbs in our modern diets are driving much of this inflammation via the immune system. By making sure that you don't consume any food product that contains more than five ingredients, you will very probably be following an anti-inflammatory diet.

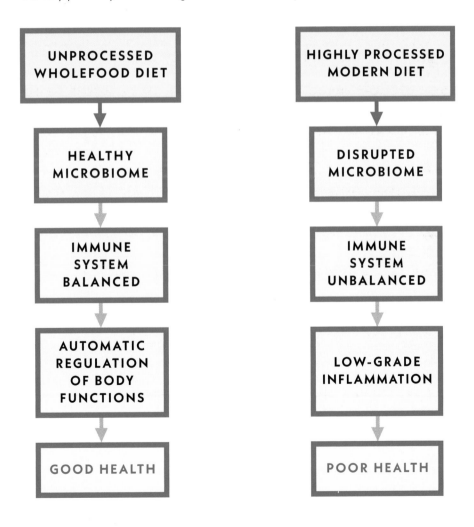

LEPTIN

And the benefits don't stop there. Another major issue I'm amazed isn't better known is that we are, in the West, increasingly resistant to the hormone leptin. It's leptin that helps make us feel full after eating. It is known as the satiety hormone.

Leptin signals to the brain that we have sufficient body fat on board as fat cells release leptin in proportion to their number. The more fat cells we have, the more leptin we produce. If leptin levels are high, the brain reduces our appetite, and may also kick in processes that burn more calories. If levels are low, the reverse happens.

This is an ancient mechanism that, when working well, keeps our body weight in check. However, like a lot of our innate biological mechanisms, it evolved in an environment very different from the highly processed food environment that we have today. Against this landscape, it has started to malfunction.

People struggling with obesity have high levels of leptin in their blood. They *should* have very little appetite, as their brain *should* be aware that their body has sufficient body fat. The problem is, the leptin is no longer effective. Their systems have become deaf to its message. They have become resistant to leptin and therefore vulnerable to overeating.

Research is ongoing into the exact mechanisms behind the development of leptin resistance but eating too much processed food and its subsequent effect on inflammation is thought to be a key factor. As we've just discovered, highly processed food causes leaky gut, which puts the immune system on high alert. When this happens, a protein called SOCS-3 is released, which can interfere with the operation of leptin. The result is unhealthy weight gain, and all the problems that come with it.

Our appetite is controlled by complex biological mechanisms in our brain and leptin plays a lead role. Leptin resistance is contributing to our collective inability to exercise control over our calories. If leptin signalling is not working well, does it really surprise you that, as a species, we are struggling? The fix for the past thirty or forty years, which has largely failed to work, is to control how much you eat and count your calories.

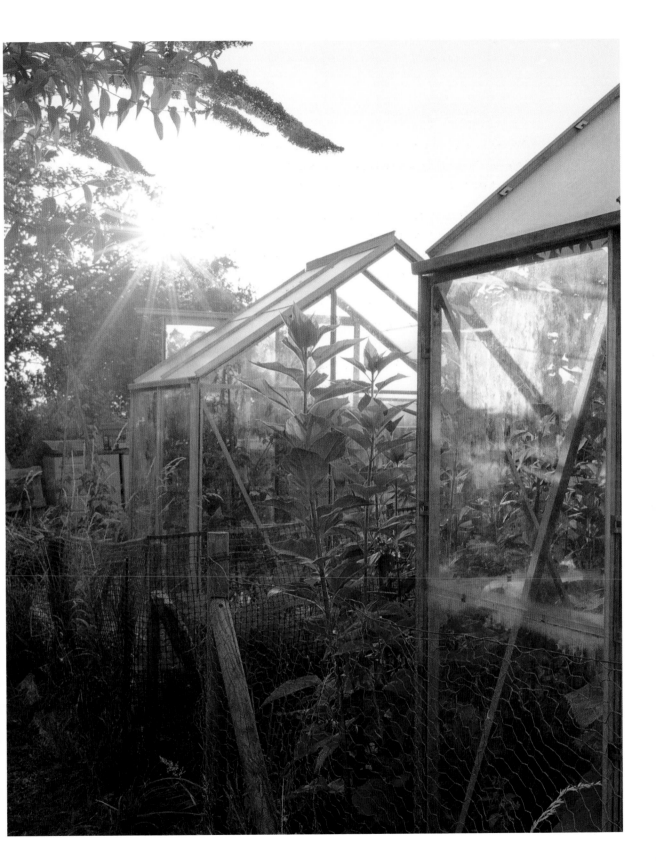

As you know by now, I don't advise this. It is not that calories are unimportant, it is just that trying to control them in the face of leptin resistance (and a 24/7 food environment) is very hard. In over sixteen years as a doctor I have *never* found this approach helpful. I prefer to reset the whole system so that your body controls calories instinctively.

(Of course, if calorie counting is working for you, I have no desire to change your behaviour – please continue!)

ANTI-INFLAMMATORY CARBS

As I have said, I don't like to demonize any one macronutrient, be it fat, carbs, sugar or whatever. Food is much more complex than its isolated parts. Very few foods in nature actually comprise just one macronutrient – the majority are made up of various combinations. Eggs contain fats, protein and carbs. Even vegetables like kale and broccoli contain carbs as well as protein. So how can you possibly remove one isolated micronutrient from your diet? You can't.

I prefer to concentrate instead on the overall value of food. And that includes carbohydrates. In his seminal 2012 paper Dr Ian Spreadbury differentiated carbs into two broad types: cellular, which are low-density carbohydrates, and acellular, which are high. High-density acellular carbs are the kind we find most often in modern processed food. They tend to be refined, highly processed and often derived from grains. Their structure has been altered. Examples include French fries, rice cakes, bagels and crisps. Dr Spreadbury argues that, because they are high in density, they cause inflammation by damaging the gut and its microbiome whilst the cellular carbs we've been eating for millennia, such as sweet potatoes, carrots and parsnips, are low density and therefore have a beneficial impact on our gut. They're also unprocessed, which means their inherent structure is intact. The carbohydrate content within them is neatly wrapped up, packaged and stored within its natural fibre coating. This means that the energy within them will be released much more slowly.

Carbohydrate density seems to be a remarkably good differentiator between ancestral 'real food' carbs and modern, highly processed acellular carbs. Spreadbury hypothesizes that the ancestral, cellular carbs we find in natural foods don't tend to drive gut microbiome disturbances and leaky gut and, therefore, don't trigger chronic inflammation.

I have many patients who do well eating moderate amounts of carbs. They lose weight and enjoy all the health benefits of any other successful health-food regime. However, they are consuming mainly healthy, cellular carbs like the Okinawans I mentioned earlier do.

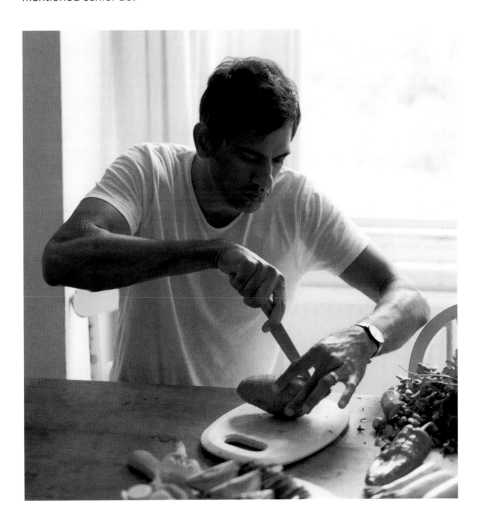

ANTI-INFLAMMATORY FATS

This same set of ideas can be applied to fats. The fats contained in highly processed foods tend to be pro-inflammatory. They can be thought of as damaged fats and include partially hydrogenated fats such as heated vegetable oils and trans-fats.

The expertise I've gained from years in clinical practice, combined with scientific research and patient feedback, has given me a definitive viewpoint. If you avoid highly refined carbohydrates and damaged processed fats, and eat an abundance of the polyphenols and antioxidants found in brightly coloured vegetables, there's no need to be overly concerned with your intake of fat. If you have unprocessed your diet, you can consume healthy, natural fats (including some saturated fat), without any problems.

More and more people are finding out for themselves that when you return your diet to foods that are minimally processed, weight, appetite and general health all seem to take care of themselves. Consciously change your diet and you unconsciously change your health.

Take a patient of mine, Semera. She'd struggled with her weight for years, trying every diet intervention you can think of. She was not only overweight but also experienced mood swings and felt tired, depressed and lacking in motivation. I told her she could eat as much as she wanted, as many times a day as she liked; the only rule was to eat only food that didn't have a high degree of processing.

I wanted Semera to avoid the ready meals, the breakfast cereals, the baked goods and muffins. These are the products made with acellular carbs. They tend to be high in energy, low in fibre and devoid of healthy polyphenols and antioxidants. To put it simply, they tend to be poor-quality 'food-like products'.

Semera had previously struggled in the kitchen. She did not enjoy cooking. She found everything around food stressful. To give her a hand, I taught her some simple, healthy meals that she could make from whole, real-food ingredients: meat, fish, eggs, nuts, seeds, fruit, plenty of vegetables, some wholegrain rice and an abundance of tasty herbs and spices.

She started feeling an improvement within days. Within one week, she had more energy, felt in a better mood and was less inclined to snack. Within one month she had lost over a stone. She said, 'Doc, I didn't know how easy this could be.' Two years on, she's never felt better. This is the hidden power of real food. I have seen this intervention alone change thousands of lives. Not only weight, but skin problems, headaches, insomnia – the list is endless.

A HACK FOR THE MODERN WORLD

No matter how closely you follow my advice to make your diet as 'minimally processed' as possible, there are going to be times when you are tempted to buy junk food. You're busy. You're working late. I know the temptations all too well. If you do succumb – or, more simply, when you have made a choice not to adhere, I have a two-part strategy that will help you recover quickly.

First of all, *don't feel guilty*. Everything we put in our mouth is a choice. Once we start assigning emotion and guilt to our food choices, we start on a slippery downward slope. Accept it as a one-off deviation, enjoy it and, if you choose to, try to make a better choice tomorrow.

Secondly, *try to limit the damage immediately*. We know that within hours of eating highly processed foods, such as kebabs and fries, we exhibit increased levels of LPS and inflammation in our bloodstream. This is remarkable. Quite literally, the food that we are eating is having a negative impact on important markers in our blood. But you can dramatically reduce (although not eliminate completely) the post-meal inflammatory response by increasing your intake of polyphenols. This is why I am so passionate about the power of the 'five a day' intervention above. The simple fact is, having some broccoli with your kebab can reduce its harmful effects. I'm not encouraging you to eat processed junk food, but I don't expect perfection, either!

OVERFED BUT UNDERNOURISHED

Of course, the benefits of eating real food don't end with its anti-inflammatory properties. Another huge problem with highly processed foods is that they're energy dense and yet nutrient poor. This probably, in part, explains why, even though obesity rates are rising, our bodies are actually becoming increasingly starved of nutrients. We are, as a society, overfed but undernourished. We're consuming copious calories and yet our cells are starving on the inside. The good news is that real food is far more nutrient dense than the stuff that comes from many of the corporations to whom we've outsourced responsibility for our collective health. By eating this way, we ensure that any calories we consume are full to the brim with nutrients.

One of the hallmark features of processed foods is the speed at which the relatively scant nutrients they do contain are absorbed into our systems. Whereas the path of broccoli can be tracked as it travels all the way down the digestive tract, dispensing different health benefits as it goes, feeding gut bugs and easing inflammation (see page 132), most processed foods are quickly and fully digested in the first few feet of the small intestine.

This is partly because most processed foods have been mechanically altered. Take bread as one simple example. In the past bread contained just three ingredients: flour, water and salt. Today, you'll struggle to find any bread, including wholegrain, in your local supermarket that has fewer than five. White bread is one of the worst culprits. Believe it or not, this stuff causes a greater sugar spike in the blood than actual table sugar! Even wholemeal bread spikes our blood sugar more rapidly than, say, a Snickers bar. As if this wasn't a big enough problem in itself, a few hours later our blood sugar then crashes back down again. When this happens, it's not only raging hunger that we feel; this crash acts as an alarm signal to the body. It fools it into thinking we're suddenly starving. Levels of the stress hormones adrenaline and cortisol soar.

We're scaring and shocking our systems in response to what we're eating. Our breakfast choices put the body into fight-or-flight mode. I have so many patients that present with what seem to be mental health issues, but who actually turn out to be reacting to unstable blood sugar levels. By cutting out processed food I can frequently stabilize their mood. Of course, I'm not saying that apparent mental health problems are always caused by diet. But I am saying that the food we eat can be a significant contributor. I've certainly seen cases where simply stabilizing blood sugar through diet led to dramatic and complete reversals. One woman had been diagnosed with chronic depression by another doctor and had come to me for a follow-up. I prescribed her an unprocessed diet that stabilized her blood sugar and, in a matter of weeks, it had completely resolved what had seemed to be her psychological problem.

She simply concentrated on eating real food. There was no magic here. There was no secret.

Surprised? You should be. Angry? You should be. Just read how food scientists writing in the journal *Public Health Nutrition* describe so much of what we're eating today:

Ultra-processed food and drink products are not modified foods, but formulations mostly of cheap industrial sources of dietary energy and nutrients plus additives using a series of processes (hence the term 'ultra-processed'). Altogether they are energy dense, high in unhealthy types of fat, refined starches, free sugars and salt, and poor sources of protein, dietary fibre and micronutrients.

We live in a society in which these food-like substances, such as commercial chocolate bars, are cheaper than an apple. How did we get here? Is it any wonder that we're struggling to maintain control of our health?

By unprocessing our diet and sticking to this simple five-ingredient rule, we can avoid so many of these problems. This is why I'm convinced that signing up to the latest food cult is not the answer. Real food is the key.

WHAT IS 'REAL FOOD' ANYWAY?

- 'Real food' is the polar opposite of modern, ultra-processed food. It is a term that I use to describe food that has traditionally been eaten by humans for millennia.

- It is minimally processed, close to its natural state and instantly recognizable – meat that looks like meat, fish that looks like fish, vegetables that look like vegetables etc.

- In contrast, most processed foods tend to be highly refined – they're in a form distinctly different from how they would appear in nature, and they tend to comprise a toxic mix of sugar, refined carbs and damaged fats whose structure has been broken in some way through processes such as being heated.

- 'Real food' reduces inflammation, nurtures a healthy microbiome and helps to educate our immune system.

14 TIPS TO UNPROCESS YOUR DIET AND EAT MORE REAL FOOD

1. Start your day with a meal containing some protein as well as some healthy, natural fat. This will help you stay full for longer, stabilize your blood sugar and help you avoid the mid-morning crash.

2. Keep an emergency snack pack with you at all times. It can live in your back-pack, your car or even your office. Mine includes a tin of wild salmon, almonds and nut butter.

3. Write a meal planner – many people find it useful to plan out their meals for the whole week so that they can plan their weekly shop.

4. Remove all highly processed food from your house – if it is not there, you are much less likely to eat it.

5. Healthy food is available to buy in every supermarket. Find out where it lives and only shop from those aisles.

6. Come up with five simple meals that you can whip up in fifteen minutes or less. These will become your go-to staples.

7. Keep frozen veggies in the house at all times. Easy to steam, they can be a quick healthy snack (especially with olive or coconut oil on top) or form part of a meal.

8. Keep pre-chopped garlic and onions in the fridge at all times.

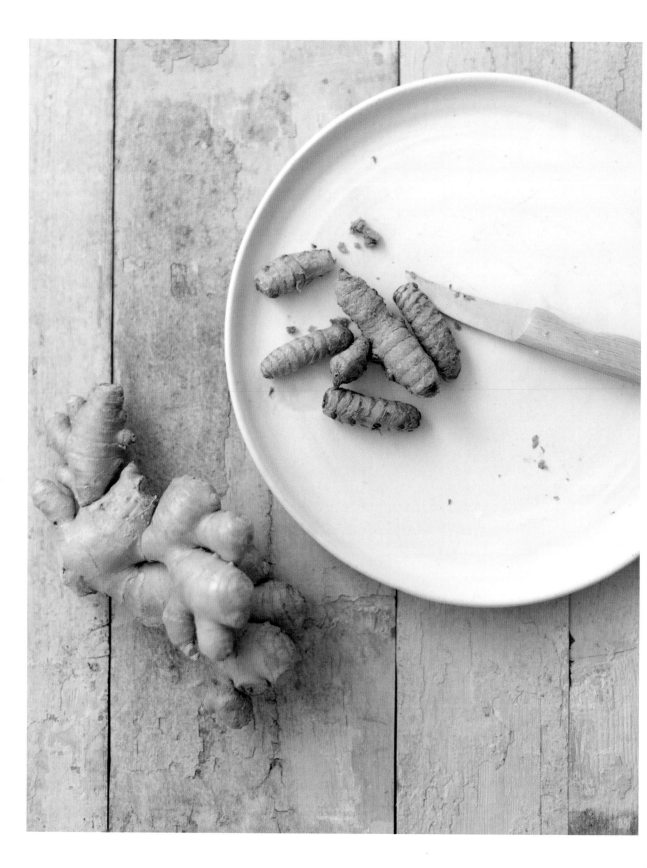

9. Make sure you always have a healthy protein source such as fish or eggs in the house. Protein is the macronutrient that keeps you most full. It takes little time to boil an egg or pan-fry a salmon fillet.

10. Why not set up an online supermarket shopping account? Once you start buying healthy foods, their marketing algorithms will propose other health foods that you may not have considered. Use this technology to help you.

11. Herbs and spices are your friends – use them freely as they are a great way to add new and exciting flavours to a meal. Many, such as turmeric, ginger and black pepper, have powerful health benefits.

12. Make your kitchen area desirable. You want to love being in your kitchen. I try to keep mine spotless and have recently bought a stereo for it so that I can listen to my favourite music whilst cooking. This helps me to unwind, switch off and enjoy cooking.

13. Reserve space in your cupboard for all the staples (nuts, sardines, fruit, veg, hummus, nut butter etc.), so you are good to go at any time.

Just remember, everything we put in our mouth is a choice. If you ever go 'off-plan', try to understand why you made that choice. You might be happy with your decision and feel that your friend's birthday party was a good enough reason to eat cake. Whatever the reason, accept it and move on. Tomorrow is another day and another opportunity to nourish your body with healthy food.

Challenge yourself to go for two weeks eating ONLY fresh, unprocessed food. Every patient of mine who has done this has always felt a difference.

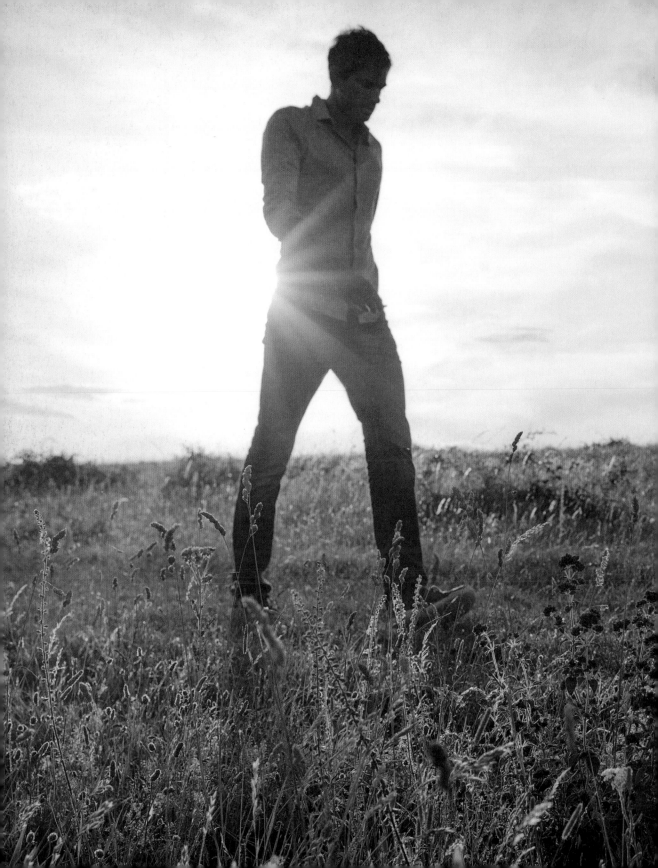

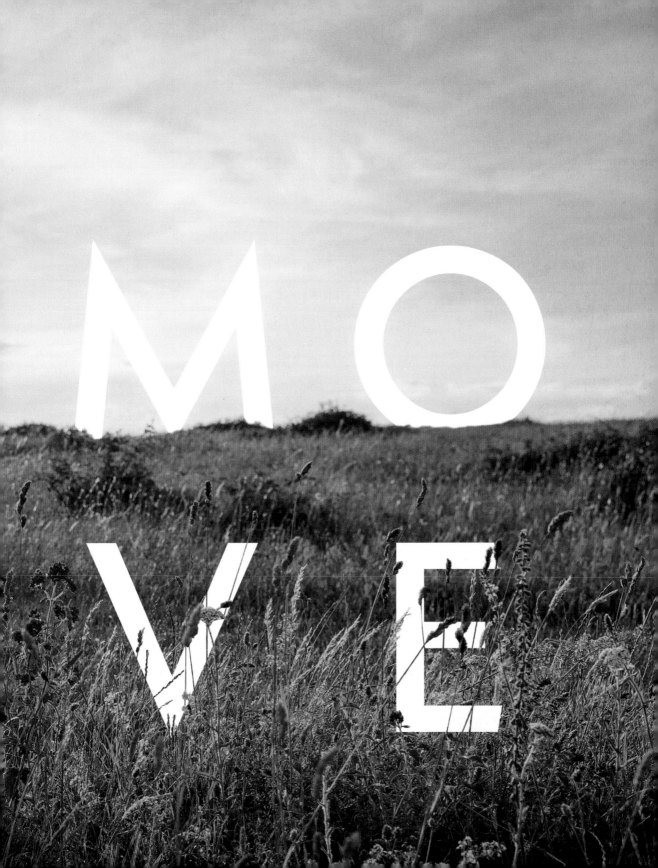

Sod calories. Sorry to be blunt, but I believe our obsession with calories is not only misguided but also actively damaging our health. It reduces the importance of food and physical activity to a simple equation and it ignores entirely the massively connected biological machine that is the human being. Health is so much more than a comparison of calories in vs energy out. And you have to ask yourself whether our cultish adherence to this dubious idea is even working anyway.

It was in the 1980s and 90s that the first 'keep fit' gurus – people like Jane Fonda and breakfast television's 'Mr Motivator', Derrick Evans – became superstars and inspired millions of Britons and Americans to try to 'get in shape'. Whilst there is no doubt they encouraged millions to get moving, the question is: Has it worked? Are we healthier than we were in 1980? Are we in better shape? Are we dying of fewer lifestyle-based diseases?

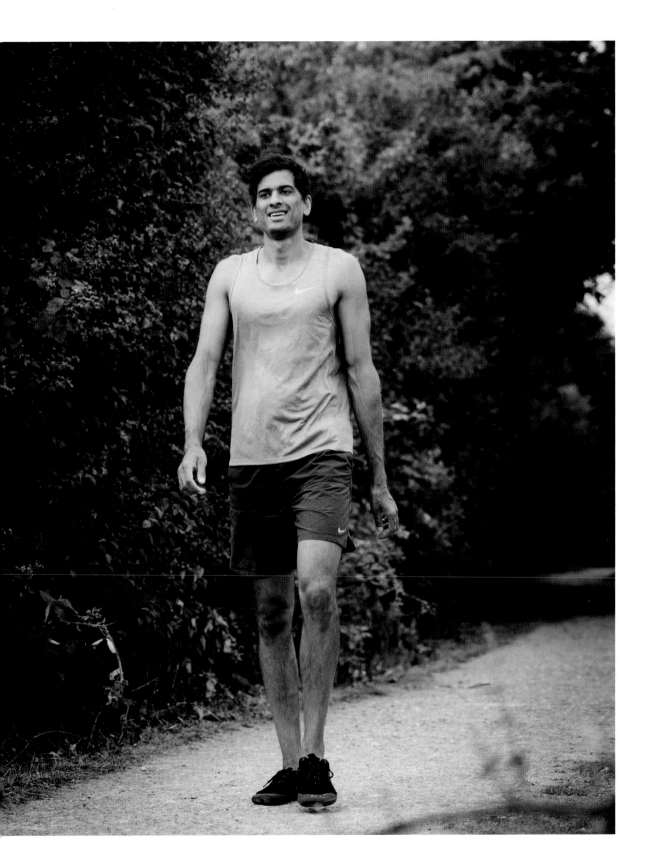

An investigation by the World Health Organization found that, in Europe and the US, 50 per cent of women and 40 per cent of men are insufficiently active, compared with South-East Asia where the figures are 15 and 19 per cent. Is it any wonder we're getting heavier and sicker with every year that passes?

I believe that our big problem with weight loss largely stems from the fact that we've been given entirely the wrong perspective on it. The keep-fit craze that emerged in the 1980s, and has since stubbornly refused to leave us, has conditioned us into seeing weight loss as the goal when, in fact, it's just a natural side-effect of living well. If we're doing enough to stay within our own personal thresholds, we don't even have to think about it. It happens automatically.

It's the same with movement. Another problem that has stemmed from the keep-fit craze is that it's conditioned us into seeing 'exercise' as a thing that happens separately from the rest of our lives. We do it at specific times of the day, scheduled alongside the household chores. We do it in special clothes. We sometimes go to a particular place that charges us lots of money to do it – and then we leave, believing our 'exercise' is now all finished until the next time and we can stop thinking about it.

ARE YOU OVERDOSING ON EXERCISE?

I think that many of us should actually cancel our gym memberships, and not necessarily for the reasons you might think. One increasing problem is that many people now, under the name of exercise, actually damage their health. Yes, it's true that as a society we don't move enough. But it's also true that some people actually need to do less. So many patients I see are feeling exhasuted, working all hours of the day, not resting properly, and then working out hard at the gym. We've all got a reserve bank of energy, and we're constantly chipping away at it and not taking the time to replenish it. If energy were money, we'd be overdrawn. That might sound glib, but growing numbers of cardiologists are convinced that there may actually be some negative effects on the heart when regularly doing endurance exercises such as marathons. A recent study involving the US army showed that extreme levels of exercise can contribute to an increase in leaky gut (see page 128). Like most things, exercise has its ideal dose. Are you overdosing?

A patient of mine, a forty-five-year-old single mother called Carina, was the chirpiest lady you've ever seen – at least on the outside. Sitting down with a slight groan, she confessed that she was feeling constantly exhausted and, even though she felt she was looking after herself extremely well, was finding it impossible to shift her excess weight. It didn't take very long for me to find out that she was running on empty. She had three energetic kids to look after and worked two jobs. Six months beforehand she'd hired a personal trainer and was hitting it hard three times per week for one full non-stop hour. These were intense sessions. She was working to the maximum every single time.

When I asked her what kind of exercises she was doing she rattled off phrases like, 'body battle', 'destroy your abs', 'killer burn'. The names alone said it all. She wasn't being helped, she was being attacked.

Whilst programmes like these can undoubtedly be helpful for someone with the time and space to recover, it just wasn't working for her. The life she led between sessions turned what could have been tough-but-good into tough-but-dangerous. It was only when she swapped the brutal personal training sessions for restorative yoga sessions that she started to lose weight.

When it comes to physical health, part of the problem is that our perceptions of what constitutes healthy behaviour are often inaccurate. The culture we live in values busyness. We use it to signify status – if we're time-poor, it means we're in demand and successful. We wear fatigue like a badge of honour. This often means squeezing that last workout in, even if we're completely spent. My social media feed is crammed with people, including many fitness professionals and doctors documenting their 6 a.m. workout despite their obvious exhaustion. Whilst their intentions are good, their message is misplaced and causing a huge amount of damage. If the life you live is already leaving you exhausted, there's simply no justification for putting yourself through the wringer in the gym. It is counterproductive. You're succeeding only in putting more and more stress on an already spent body. You may get a temporary boost of endorphins, but at what cost?

THE WORLD IS YOUR GYM

Another reason I think many of us should be cancelling our gym memberships is that it's much better for us to see our whole lives as a potential workout. We need to stop thinking about getting our exercise chore done and start thinking about making it a part of our daily lives. In fact, I believe we should stop talking about 'exercise' altogether and start thinking, instead, about 'movement'. We simply need to move more during the day, throughout the day, every day. We need to design our lives around movement. We're designed to be active, but modern life makes us sit for hours in cars on the commute and chains us to a desk for eight hours. One 2010 study that examined sitting as an emerging health risk found that many adults spend 70 per cent of their day in a seat, whilst the other 30 per cent involved doing only light activity. Another expert, Dr James Levine of the Mayo Clinic in Rochester, has gone so far as to state that 'sitting is a lethal activity'. We wouldn't expect this level of routine inactivity in zoo animals, but we accept it of ourselves. The time has come for us to admit it's just not working for us. In fact, it's killing us. Physical inactivity is one of the biggest causes of premature death. According to the World Health Organization it accounts for 5 per cent of all the deaths in the world. It's a greater health risk than being overweight or obese. Other studies have suggested that it can be as bad for us as smoking.

Whether inactivity is really as bad as smoking, I'm not sure – and quite frankly, I am not sure it really matters. The uncomfortable truth is that prolonged sitting is far more problematic for health than is generally realized. The most compelling link comes from studies that look at those who watch television. TV time is strongly correlated with an increase in type 2 diabetes, cardiovascular disease and all-cause mortality. At the moment, this is just an association, so we have to be careful – it's not been shown that sitting is the cause of these problems and it's probably only part of the whole picture (prolonged TV time is also associated with unhealthy dietary choices, junk food advertising, less time spent doing other activities, etc.). But, that said, do these results really surprise you?

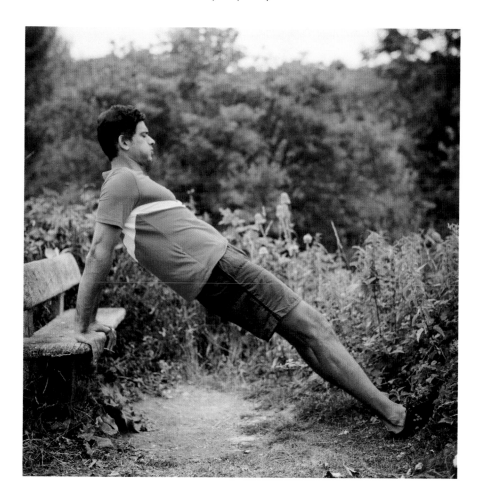

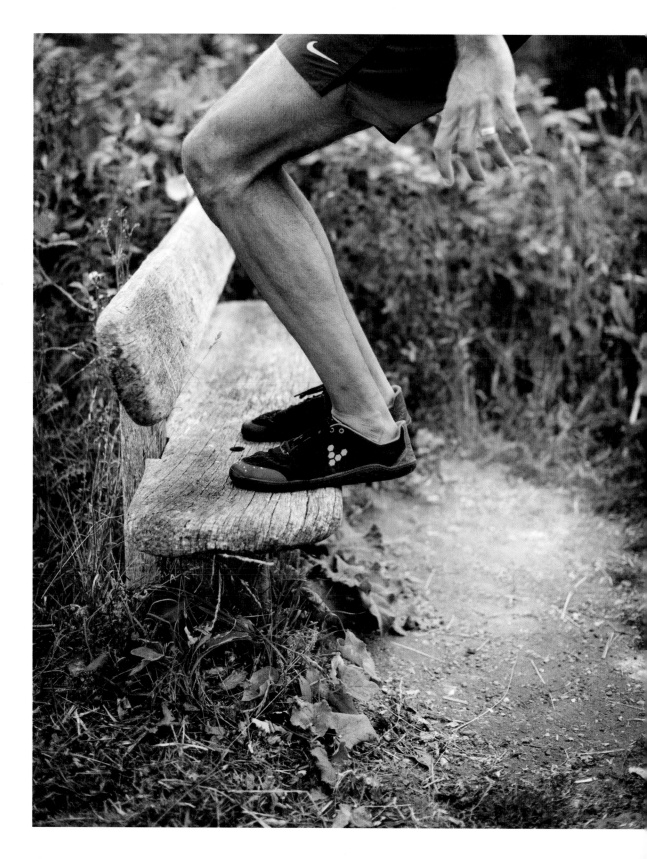

Further studies have found that we simply can't undo the damage that prolonged sitting does to us by going to a spinning or gym class for forty-five minutes after work. But there's good news too. A 2017 study by researchers in the Netherlands found that breaking up all that sitting with light activities had significant improvements over and beyond the kind of structured exercise programme we'd get at the gym. According to the study's authors, 'Breaking sitting with standing and light-intensity walking effectively improved twenty-four-hour glucose levels and improved insulin sensitivity in individuals with type 2 diabetes to a greater extent than structured exercise.' A gym session is not the antidote to sitting, then. The answer is to sit less and spend more time fidgeting and moving. Design your day around it.

It's partly exciting, cutting-edge findings such as these that have honed my movement interventions. These interventions have myriad health benefits and, as always, a direct impact on all the other pillars. For example, movement and exercise improve your immune system functioning by increasing the activity of 'natural killer' cells: immune cells that fight infection. They also improve mitochondrial biogenesis, which is the creation of new mitochondria that enhances the ability of our bodies to make energy (see box on page 111). They even change the composition of our gut microbiota. They reduce inflammation, reduce oxidative stress, regulate hormonal dysfunction and improve blood pressure as well as circulatory and lymphatic flow around the body. Regular walking is also one of the best things you can do to prevent Alzheimer's.

All five of the following interventions will improve your health but if I had to prioritize just one to get you started, it would be the first. The benefits of getting your 10,000 steps per day are profound. Not only that, but if you tackle this one successfully, you'll find the other four much easier to take on.

1. WALK MORE

Aim for at least 10,000 steps per day.

This first intervention is deceptively simple. I'm the first to admit that walking 10,000 steps a day is a completely arbitrary goal. It's also true that you can't out-walk a bad diet – if you're eating the wrong things, no amount of strolling can reverse the damage you're doing to yourself. However, this is a good simple rule to set us in the direction of being more active. For many, walking is a gateway exercise that is the start of the journey from not moving at all to optimal movement. Walking, like breathing, is such a fundamental process that it's one of the core activities that the brain does without the need for conscious control.

Benefits include:

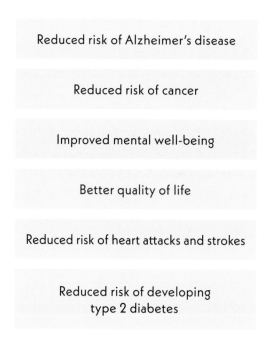

Reduced risk of Alzheimer's disease

Reduced risk of cancer

Improved mental well-being

Better quality of life

Reduced risk of heart attacks and strokes

Reduced risk of developing
type 2 diabetes

I know that 10,000 sounds like an awful lot of steps, but it's less than you might think. I see people in my practice who do almost nothing in the day and yet still manage to rack up a couple of thousand. In fact, 1,000 steps is only about ten minutes on your feet. If you can walk without much discomfort, you can achieve it. In fact, it's achievable for almost every single patient that walks through my door, whether they are twenty years old or eighty. If you can afford it, buy a Fitbit or keyring pedometer. These keep track of your steps and mean you can also leave your smartphone at home, which in turn means you can enjoy your walk in peace without the bombardment of texts, emails and social media alerts.

And it's not hard to find the opportunities either. Make it a rule that you never sit down for more than one hour at a time. Put a reminder on your computer or get your Fitbit to buzz you every sixty minutes and, if you haven't stood up, go to the drinks machine or to the toilet. What about taking the stairs instead of the lift? I pretty much never take lifts, unless I'm staying near the top of a high-rise hotel. At airports, I always take the stairs. They're usually empty, whilst the escalators are rammed full of people. It sometimes (although not all the time) takes a bit longer, but saving time to harm your health isn't a good deal for me.

What about when you're going to work or into town? Do you have to get the bus to your nearest stop? Why not get off two or three stops early and walk the rest? Do you have to park at the space that's closest to the supermarket's entrance, or as close as possible to your destination? My own family has made it a rule to walk to school and back every day. We live 0.7 miles away, so this gets me 3,000 steps in before the day has even kicked off. If I manage to be around for pick-up too, that's 6,000 steps just from doing the school run. When you start seeing the whole world as your gym, you start seeing all the opportunities you have to make moving a simple and achievable part of your daily life.

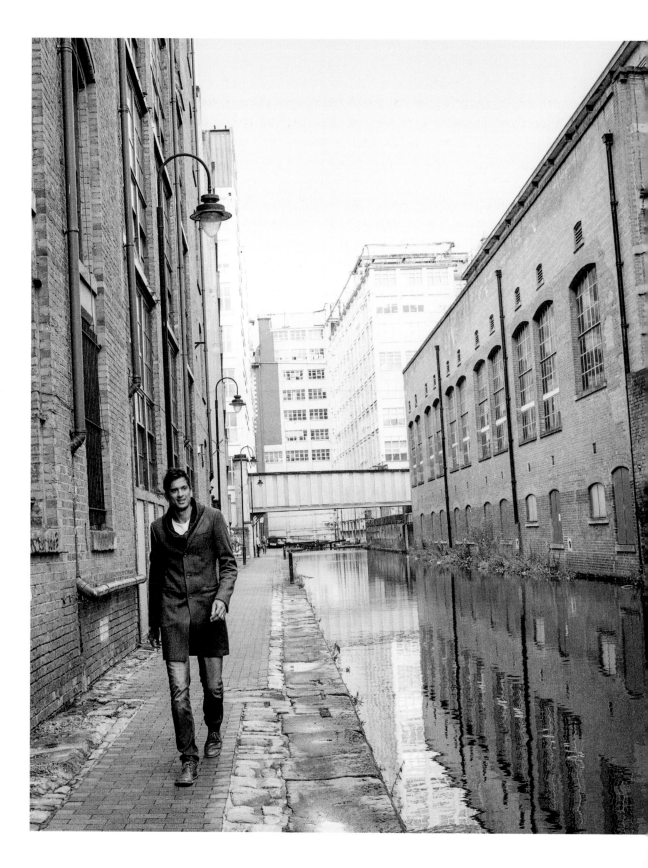

At work, I'm one of the few doctors who don't use the tannoy system. I don't use it for several reasons. Partly, I think it's more polite to go to the waiting room, greet my patients and shake their hand. But it's also an excuse to get more steps in. If I've got forty-five patients to see in a day then I'm getting in and out of my chair forty-five times over six or seven hours. At my previous practice in Oldham, I'd be out of my chair every ten minutes, walk twenty seconds down to reception, greet the patient and walk twenty seconds back. That added up to nearly half an hour of walking, or 3,000 steps, just by making that one change.

What can you do in your own life that builds in this movement? Why not walk across your office to talk to your colleague rather than sending an email? How about taking the stairs instead of the lift? Have you ever sent a family member or partner a text inside your own house rather than telling them something in person? How crazy is that?

GO FOR A MORNING STROLL

A bonus tip would be to do as much of your walking as possible in the morning. One recent study found that exposure to bright morning light correlates with a lower body weight. This makes perfect sense to me, as it fits with what we know about the body's natural circadian rhythms (see pages 112, 214). Exposure to light is a primary mechanism for getting our internal rhythms set properly and making sure they're working well. Getting outside in the morning is also one of the interventions in the Sleep pillar, so why not kill two birds with one stone?

2. BECOME STRONGER

Do some form of strength training twice a week.

Muscle is the forgotten organ. And, make no mistake, it is an organ. We tend to think of muscle as nothing more than dumb meat that's simply there to power our limbs, but it plays any number of active roles in the daily running of our bodies. Here's just one example: our muscle controls not only the way in which hormones are released into our bodies but also how they're regulated. The more we have of it, the better able we are to control the action of those hormones. All of our cells contain mitochondria (see page 111), and our muscle cells have a particularly high concentration. Mitochondria are our energy factories. Therefore the more muscle we have, the more mitochondria we have, so the more potential we have to make energy.

When we're strength training, with every single muscle contraction we make, our body releases a variety of chemical messengers called cytokines, one of which, interleukin 6, is of critical importance because in this context it switches off inflammation. Every single muscle contraction we make is an anti-inflammatory signal to the body. We've already talked about just how common and how devastating a problem inflammation can be – and that long-term, unresolved inflammation is a key driver of almost every single modern disease we have. Strength training and high-intensity interval training, which we will come to shortly (or, ideally, a combination of the two), helps turn it off.

More muscle also means more insulin receptors. In other words, the more muscle you have, the more space your insulin has to put all the food you're taking in. Think of it as like having bigger cupboards. More room in there means you can get away with eating more junk (though this is not what I am recommending!), and that makes you less likely to develop type 2 diabetes.

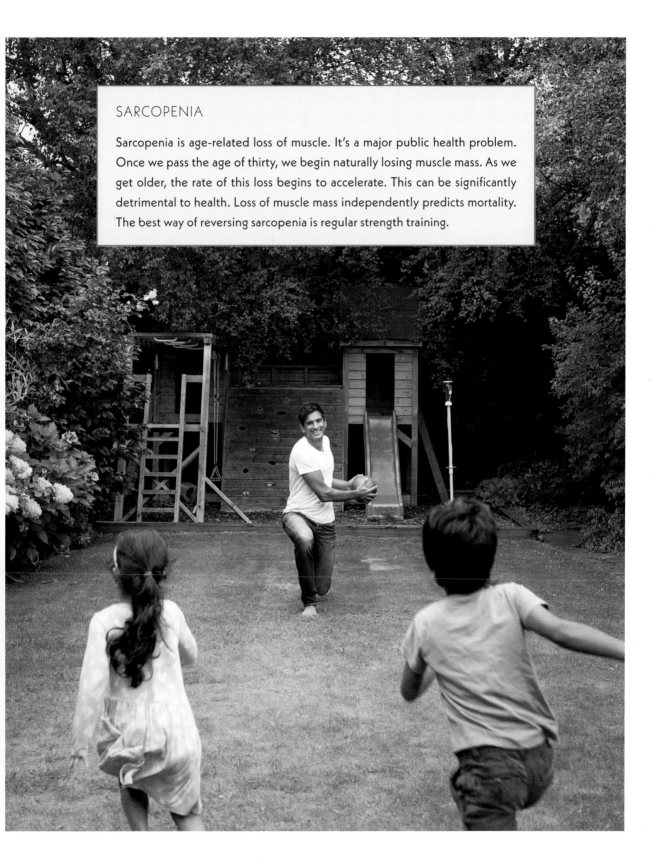

SARCOPENIA

Sarcopenia is age-related loss of muscle. It's a major public health problem. Once we pass the age of thirty, we begin naturally losing muscle mass. As we get older, the rate of this loss begins to accelerate. This can be significantly detrimental to health. Loss of muscle mass independently predicts mortality. The best way of reversing sarcopenia is regular strength training.

BENEFITS OF STRENGTH TRAINING

Strength training has many benefits, including:

Better body composition

Increased self-esteem

Reversed ageing

Reduced risk of type 2 diabetes, cardiovascular disease and stroke

Better insulin sensitivity

Improved brain health

Reduced risk of muscle loss

Reduced risk of osteoporosis

Improved hormonal profile

Reduction in stress and anxiety

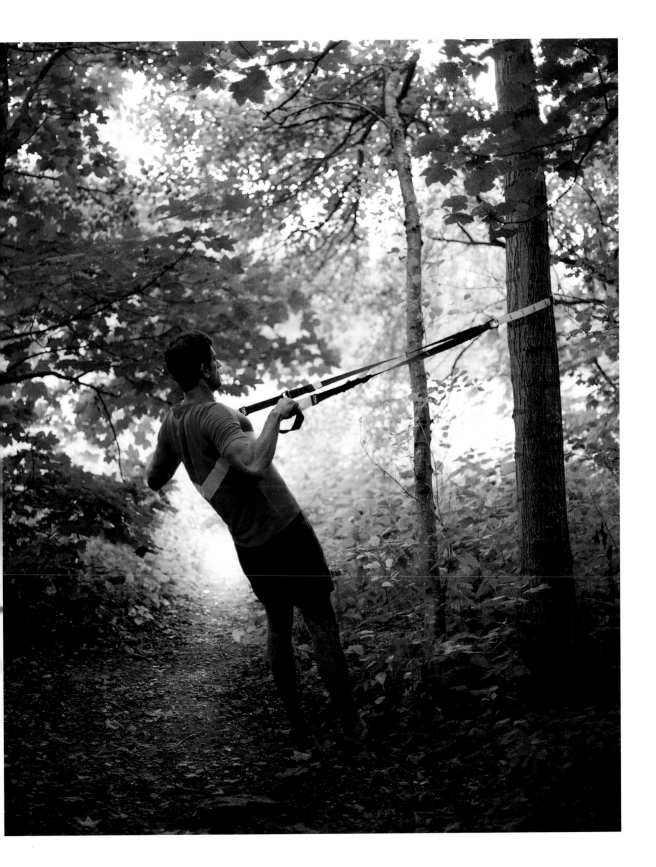

REVERSING AGEING

Research suggests that having more muscle is self-reinforcing – the more muscle you have, the more muscle you maintain. It also has a large influence on how strong your bones are. Strength training has been proven to reverse ageing in human skeletal muscles. This is especially important for people who are middle aged and older. Our perception is that teenagers and twenty-somethings are the ones who are pumping iron to get all buff-looking, but we urgently need to shift our perception. Above the age of thirty, if we're physically inactive we lose up to 3 to 5 per cent of our muscle mass every decade. Between the ages of fifty and sixty, muscle power declines by around 3 per cent each year. This is an extremely serious problem, because loss of muscle mass is a strong predictor of late-life mortality. When muscle loss becomes problematic we call it 'sarcopenia', and rates of this disorder increase linearly with age. Current estimates have it that up to 15 per cent of people sixty-five years and older, and as many as half of all eighty-somethings, are suffering with it.

Like most things in the body, the causes of sarcopenia are many. It's often seen in people who are inactive, but another of the factors that contribute to it is the inability of our muscles to regenerate after injury. Strength training increases the production of different types of muscle fibres, which help to rejuvenate damaged muscle, which is yet another way it helps us avoid sarcopenia. It also helps increase cognitive performance and there's evidence, too, that it might go some way towards preventing Alzheimer's.

There's even been some exciting academic work suggesting that strength training actually changes the way people think. The scientists compared women who did aerobic exercise versus women who did strength training (although there's no reason to believe this effect is gender specific). Both groups showed an improvement in elements of their 'executive brain function', which alludes to such things as their working memory and their ability to modify behaviour in response to a changing situation. But the strength-training group gained something extra. They were the only ones who experienced improved powers of attention. They were even found to be better at resolving conflicts.

I could go on listing benefits for ever. But the point is that strength training is undervalued and underutilized across all ages and of critical importance once we get over the age of thirty. We simply must do some form of strength training every week to maintain muscle mass, muscle function and our ability to use our brains. One of the reasons we don't is that we've overcomplicated our ideas of fitness. We don't have to go to a gym or dress up in special clothing (although you can if you want to) – we can do it in our kitchen in our usual daywear (see page 166).

Try and find a type of strength training that you enjoy. That is the *only* way that you will not only start, but continue doing it twelve months later. Cycling has exploded in popularity in recent years and can be a great option for some. Indoor climbing is another option that helps promote mindfulness at the same time. Yoga can also serve as strength training and other benefits include increased mobility and enhanced relaxation.

Some of you, no doubt, will love the gym and getting started with a personal trainer can be a fantastic motivating tool. But if you don't have the finances or easy access to one, don't let that be an excuse. The body is a heavy weight – use it!

FIVE-MINUTE KITCHEN WORKOUT

I created this workout to help my patients fit in their strength training around their busy lives. It has become a huge hit with many of my patients. I consulted with a couple in their 60s who had let their physical health go. I modified this workout to suit their ability levels. Although being initially sceptical, within weeks what had started in their kitchen ended up on their upstairs landing and they were doing the whole sequence 5 nights a week whilst running their bath.

Use the following instructions as a guide but feel free to change as you see fit. To start, aim to do this workout twice a week. The secret is to start slowly and build up.

1. 5–10 squats – Aim to go down as far as you can whilst keeping your back upright and your feet flat on the ground. Hold on to the kitchen worktop for support, if needed.

2. 5–10 calf raises – Whilst standing straight, move on to your tiptoes as high as you can. Hold on to a door or worktop if you need support.

3. 5–10 press-ups – Place your hands wider than shoulder width apart and lower your chest down between them before pushing back up again. Start against a wall then, as you get stronger, against a kitchen worktop; eventually you will be able to do them on the floor.

4. 5–10 triceps dips – Place your hands on a worktop, a chair or the floor. Lower yourself whilst bending your elbows behind you. Modify your hand position depending on ability: on the worktop is easiest and on the floor, the hardest.

5. 5–10 lunges – Put one leg forwards and bend at the knee. Keep your torso upright and hold on for support as required. As you become stronger you can add in a side rotation. Make sure you do both legs.

See drchatterjee.com for full video instructions.

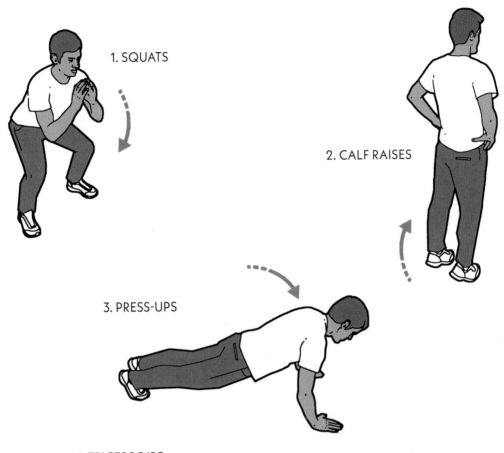

1. SQUATS

2. CALF RAISES

3. PRESS-UPS

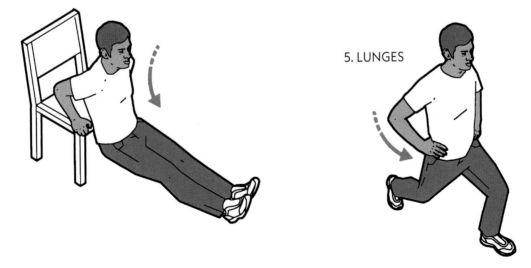

4. TRICEPS DIPS

5. LUNGES

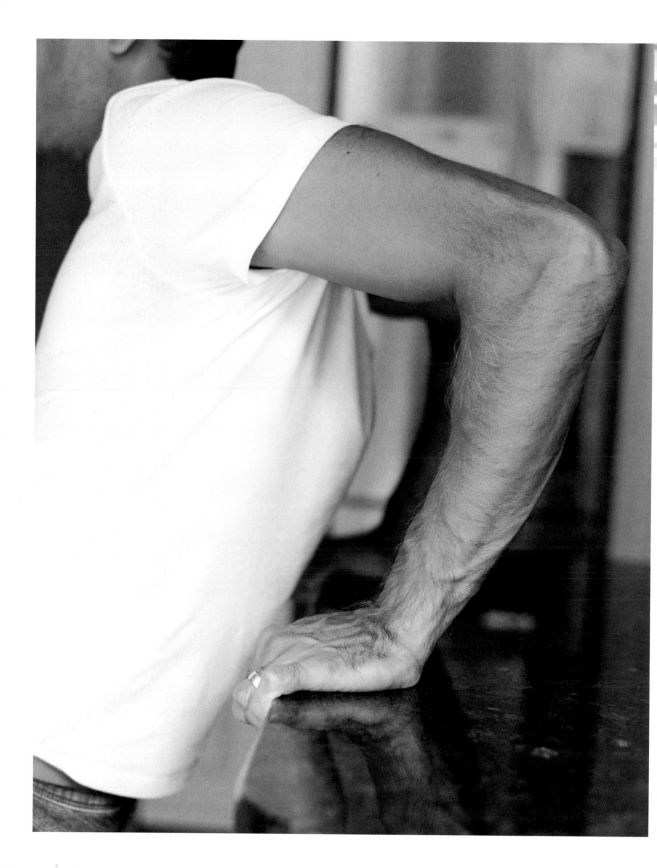

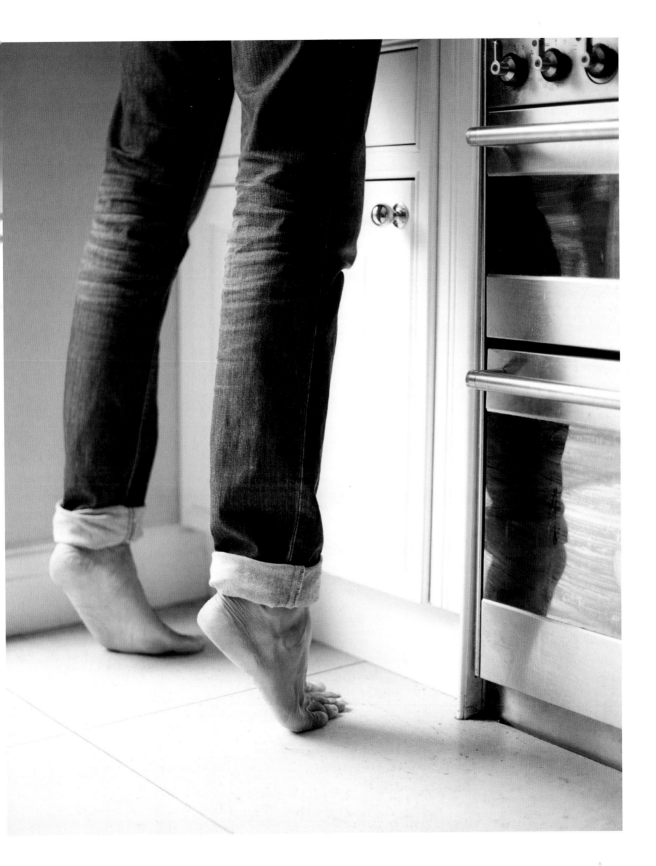

3. BEGIN REGULAR HIGH-INTENSITY INTERVAL TRAINING

Find a form of HIIT that works for you and do two ten-minute sessions each week.

What if I told you it was possible to exercise less and achieve more? Would you believe me? Or would you think I was hawking some too-good-to-be true 'wellness' scheme and was about to ask you to buy a £600 gadget and sign some byzantine contract? The amazing fact of the matter is, a lot of modern science is telling us exactly that. High-intensity interval training – often shortened to HIIT – is a very specific form of training that's been shown to have some fantastic health benefits. In simple terms, it refers to exercising hard, but in short bursts.

Health benefits include:

Slowing the ageing process

Losing dangerous, internal visceral fat (see page 174)

Increasing the growth of brain cells

Increasing mitochondrial numbers and function

Improving insulin sensitivity, which helps prevent type 2 diabetes

Losing weight

Back in my early days as a GP, I used to stop at the gym on the way to work. I needed to be at my desk by 7.30 to start going through paperwork, blood results and all the other important but time-consuming items that pile up on a doctor's desk before they even start seeing patients. I'd leave my house at 6.20 to ensure I'd be at the gym when it opened at 6.30. It would take me about five minutes to check in, change and get to the equipment. From 6.35 until 6.55 I'd work out, jumping from side to side, sprinting on the squash court, lunging up and down the gym and maybe finishing off with some weights. By 7.10 I was back in my work clothes, freshly shaved and showered. I'd arrive at my surgery at about 7.25 and was ready to go with my computer all set up at 7.30.

One of my colleagues at the surgery said to me, 'What's the point of just going for twenty minutes? You may as well not bother.' She was a GP and this was her strong belief. In fact, she was someone who used to battle with her weight and always found the gym a struggle. She'd only go when she had a full hour to dedicate to it, otherwise she felt she was wasting her time. This was a big mistake. And yet I see it being made every day by friends, colleagues and patients. The fact is, you do not need to dedicate all that much time to working out.

Whether you're spending too much time in the gym or not enough, HIIT could be the answer. The difference between HIIT and a traditional exercise session is that, rather than going non-stop for an extended period of time, your workout is sectioned off into lots of smaller sessions, with 'intervals' of rest in between them. And these sessions must be intense. By that I mean they should be intense for you. I want you to be pushing yourself. You should go all out, sweat running, heart pumping. By the end, you should be out of breath and unable to hold a conversation for a good thirty seconds. This sounds tough, but it's important to remember that you only have to do this for a short period of time. You'll feel recovered again pretty quickly.

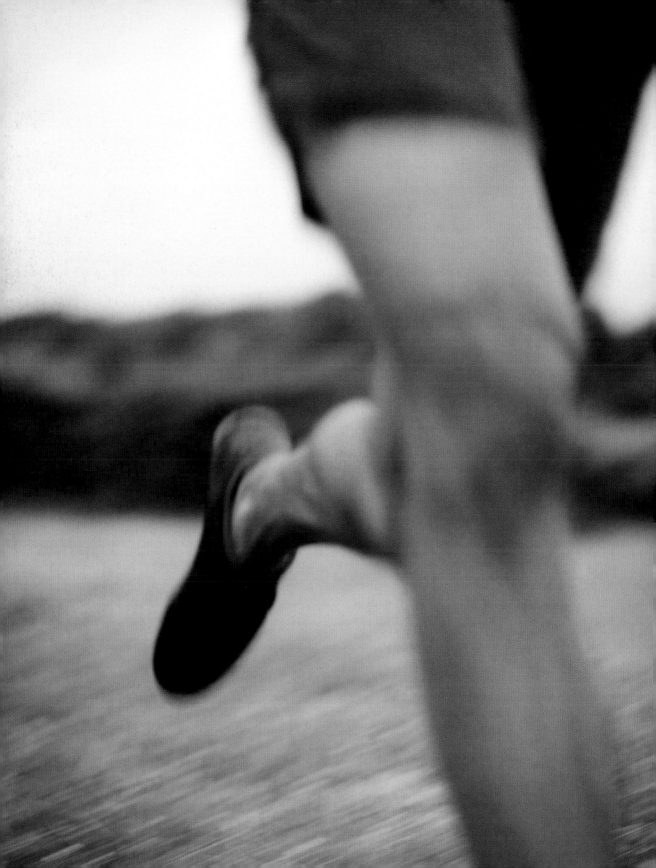

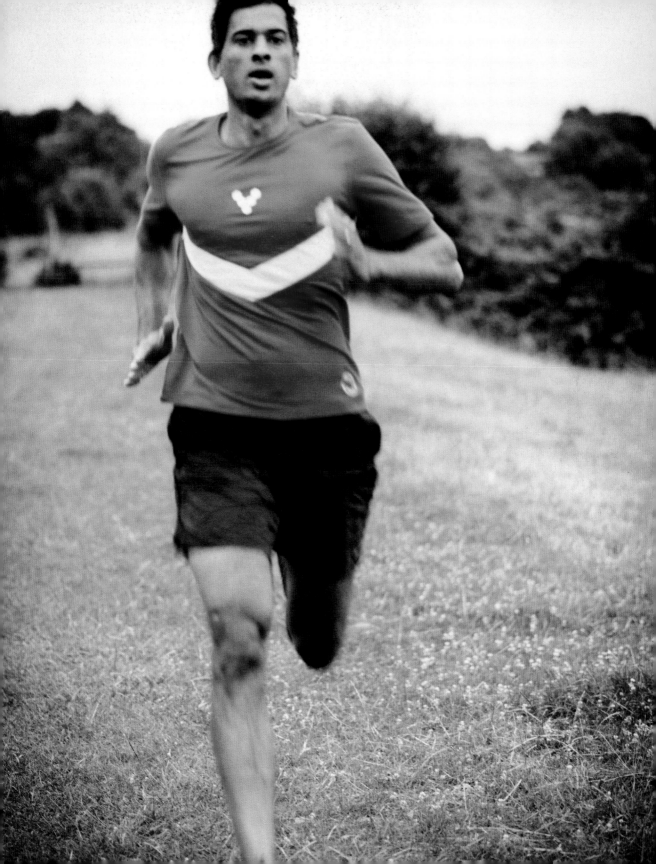

The evidence that the body responds better to this form of training is powerful and growing. One recent study found that an eleven-minute HIIT workout gives as much benefit as one hour of continuous activity. Another, by one of the world's leading researchers into HIIT, Martin Gibala, showed that one minute of intense working out, pushing yourself as hard as you possibly can in three twenty-second bursts of intense cycling spread out over ten minutes, showed equivalent improvement to forty-five minutes of moderate-intensity cycling. Think about these numbers for a moment. They're truly incredible. It's surely little wonder the famous journalist A. A. Gill once wondered if HIIT could be 'the most time saving invention since the microwave'.

Just as impressive are the positive threshold effects that HIIT has on our massively connected bodies. HIIT improves our insulin sensitivity much more than ordinary forms of exercise, making us less likely to contract type 2 diabetes. It improves our mitochondrial function, which enables all bodily processes to work better. It reduces inflammation. It makes our blood vessels work more efficiently. It increases cardiorespiratory fitness. It's really good for weight loss. The very latest research on HIIT is even hinting that it might slow the ageing process. Researchers from the Mayo Clinic published a study in March 2017 which found that HIIT may reverse ageing at the cellular level.

VISCERAL FAT

And that's not all. There are lots of different types of fat in the human body that are classified not only by their actual structure but also by where they're found. One particularly dangerous kind is called 'visceral fat'. People can look as if they don't have a weight problem, but when you put them in a scanner, you discover that they have layers of internal fat covering their organs. This is visceral fat. People sometimes refer to sufferers of the condition as TOFI – 'thin on the outside, fat on the inside'. Just because you look thin, it doesn't necessarily follow that you are thin. What's more, visceral fat is more dangerous than what we call 'subcutaneous' fat, which is the stuff that lies just beneath the skin. It puts you at increased risk of heart attack and stroke. And guess what? HIIT is especially good at getting rid of visceral fat.

BUILDING BRAIN HEALTH

What about brain health? We know all kinds of exercise are helpful for our cognition, but one 2015 study found that HIIT helps increase something called 'brain-derived neurotrophic factor' or BDNF. BDNF is a supportive molecule for the brain. Think of it like high-octane fuel. It helps prevent terrible brain disorders such as dementia. It grows new nerve cells. Another study showed that just twenty minutes of aerobic exercise a day can increase BDNF as well as the growth of cells in the hippocampus, which is the part of your brain responsible for memory. There's no pharmaceutical drug that can increase BDNF and, if there were, everyone on earth would want it. And yet movement can do this – especially HIIT.

But which particular form of exercise increases BDNF the most? This – at least at the moment – is very hard to say. However, one exciting study showed that following intense, rather than low-intensity, exercise, people not only learned vocabulary 20 per cent faster but also had bigger spikes in their BDNF levels. Could there be an additional benefit for HIIT? I think so.

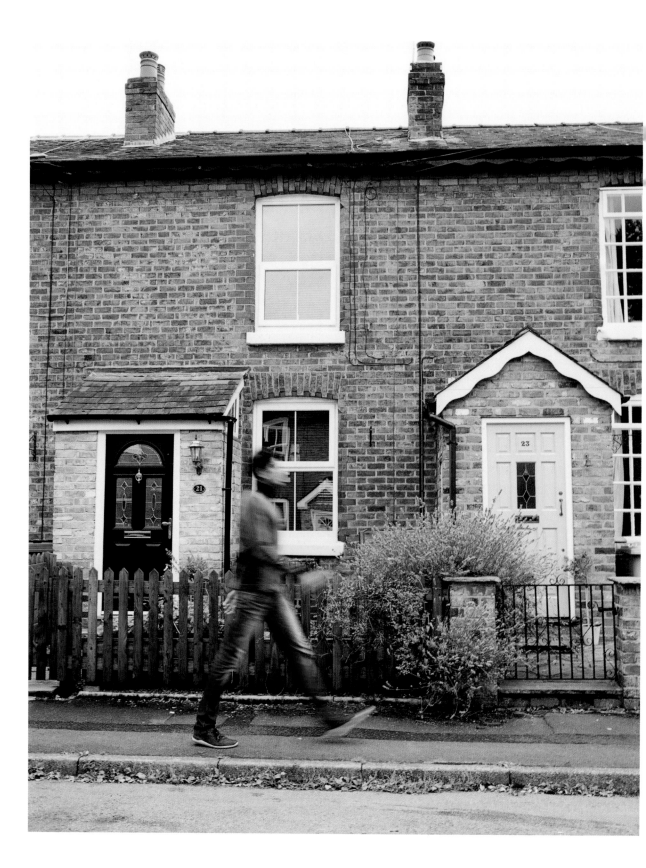

CHOOSING THE WORKOUT THAT WORKS FOR YOU

There are a lot of different versions of HIIT, but I like to think of it as any form of exercise in which there's a sudden change in activity that forces your body to adapt. It must be a period of high-intensity movement followed by a period of low-intensity movement.

And it must be 'intense' as perceived by you. My aim with this book is to help you simplify health. This is why I don't want you measuring your pulse or counting your breathing rate. As long as you perceive it as very hard, it works for me. For example, if you like going to the gym, you can jump on a treadmill and do forty seconds at perhaps twelve kilometres per hour (or whatever pace feels very hard to you), then, for one minute and twenty seconds, go at four kilometres per hour, which will be much easier. That sharp change forces your body to adapt physiologically. Doing it in bursts gives you much more benefit for your buck. Repeat this three to five times.

But it doesn't have to be that hard. It all depends upon your current fitness levels. It doesn't even have to be in a gym. One of my most popular workouts (featured in the first series of my BBC show, *Doctor in the House*) is one of the simplest. Many of my patients love it for the ease with which it fits into their everyday life. It works like this. Walk out of your front door and go to the end of your road. From there, walk as fast as you can for one minute. When that minute's over, look to see which house number you've arrived at, then walk at a normal pace back to the start. Now you repeat the same sequence, but this time you want to see if you can beat yourself and get to a house further down the road. This may sound relatively easy, but by the time you have done this three times, you will be really feeling it. Try and do this five times altogether. It will only take you ten or fifteen minutes maximum, you don't need a gym membership or fancy clothes and the benefits are profound.

Don't want to go outside on a rainy October day? Fine. How about doing ten burpees, ten star jumps and ten side lunges sequentially in your living room for forty seconds? Then spend the next eighty seconds walking around slowly and then repeat five times. Alternatively, try a combination of fast alternating leg lunges, press-ups and kettlebell swings. If none of these appeal, make up your own. There are infinite possibilities!

4. MOVEMENT SNACKING

Make a habit of doing three or four 'movement snacks'
five days a week.

One of my favourite quotes is from George Bernard Shaw, who said, 'We don't stop playing because we grow old; we grow old because we stop playing.' This is all too true and I've no doubt that one of the reasons we find our health and energy levels deteriorating (and thus put on weight) as we grow older is that we're no longer running around having fun – playing tag, kicking a ball about, skipping in the playground. I'd love it if it became the norm among us grown-up children that we rediscovered this part of our nature, which becomes repressed as all the responsibilities of adulthood pile in and weigh us down. Imagine if, in offices up and down the country, everyone did a two-minute workout together before they went out for lunch! Some quick lunges, dips, air squats or side lunges would be amazing for company team-building and morale and even better for the nation's health.

This intervention is focused on fun and play. One of the reasons people who engage in sport tend to stick with their regimes so well is because they're doing it for pleasure. I've recently rediscovered the joy I find in playing squash. I get to unwind, engage my competitive side and, by default, I work up a sweat and improve my health. Not only that, I also feel fantastic afterwards. I play with one of my primary school buddies and it's not unusual for us to just spend the first ten minutes laughing and taking the mick out of each other. Those forty-five minutes are golden for me. I simply cannot wait for my weekly game.

PLAYING TOGETHER

Doing our movement snacks in company really helps, whether it's with your partner, your friends or your fellow workers. And it doesn't have to be something long and intense like a game of squash. What I'm really talking about here is little bite-sized snacks of movement. Grab a skipping rope, do a load of star jumps or race your colleagues around the office. When I am at home, I will dive onto the floor (or go in the garden) and mimic various animal moves with the kids; an ape, a bear, a frog or a crab. Fun as well as energizing – it leaves us all breathless. We change it up every day but it could be squats, primal tag (see below), step-ups on the stairs . . . Sometimes we just put some music on and start singing and dancing. It drives my wife crazy but we have a complete laugh. By the time we start eating dinner, we're often a little out of breath. The fantastic thing about doing these movement snacks before eating is that they actually change the way your body deals with your meal. Several studies have shown that when you do some exercise immediately before food, your blood sugar rises less after you've eaten.

One of my favourite games was introduced to me by a friend called Darryl Edwards, creator of the Primal Play Method. He calls it Primal Play Tag. You need two people and the aim is simply to try to touch your opponent between the knee and the hip. So you're both simultaneously trying to avoid and trying to tag. This is three-dimensional movement. You can do it pretty much anywhere, and it's so much fun that you just don't feel like you're exercising.

THE KITCHEN GYM

For me, the kitchen has always been a fantastic place to indulge in a quick movement snack. I remember as a teenager, I'd use the two minutes it took for my food to warm up in the microwave to hit the deck and bang out some press-ups. Nowadays, I do twenty squats with my kids in the time it takes for spinach to steam. You could take two bottles of olive oil and lift them up over your head and to the sides, hop on each leg for thirty seconds or even simply jump from side to side. The point is to get your heart pumping three or four times a day – but it has to be fun!

THE OFFICE WORKOUT

I'd love it to become the norm in offices around the UK to have a little play-based movement snack at the start of lunch every day. You could do a combination of the movements mentioned below or devise your own. How about starting every lunch break with the following? Dare as many of your colleagues as you can to join in:

1. Five triceps dips on your desk (see triceps dips on page 166)

2. Five star jumps

3. Five hand clap lunges on each leg – Stand opposite a partner and do a lunge towards each other. As you do, use your left hand to do a high five with their left hand.

4. Five side lunges on each leg – Step to the left. Keep your body facing forward and your right foot planted on the floor, whilst bending your left knee.

5. Five desk press-ups (see press-ups on page 166)

This is meant to be fun. No judgement. No competition. Just a way of engaging everyone to be active. The great thing about doing this as a group is that it is much more likely to become permanent. Some days you won't feel like doing it but your colleagues will. Hopefully, that will be the motivation to do this every day at work! It's easy to fall into the trap of thinking that small bursts of movement like these won't have much effect, but it's these little things you do every day that translate into the big health outcomes. The truth is, good health isn't meant to be that hard, nor, is it meant to be boring.

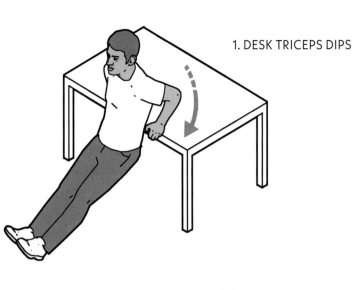

1. DESK TRICEPS DIPS

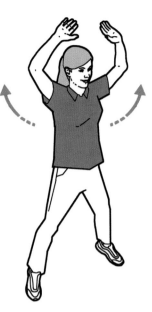

2. STAR JUMPS

3. PARTNER LUNGES

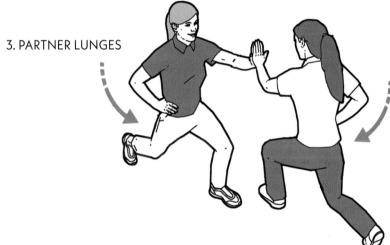

5. DESK PRESS-UPS

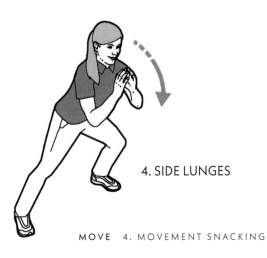

4. SIDE LUNGES

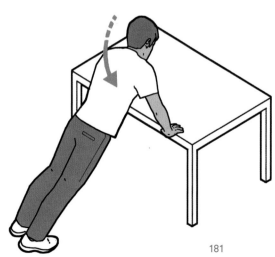

5. WAKE UP YOUR SLEEPY GLUTES

Do at least one glute movement every day, and the whole series four times per week.

Would you build your house on shaky foundations? Would you teach your kids to construct their Lego creations on a sloping floor? Would you stack Jenga blocks on jelly? Well, that's the sort of thing I see many people doing these days with their bodies. Because of modern life, our basic movement mechanics simply aren't working any more. We spend our days in bent-over postures and our bodies adapt. We mould into the shapes in which we spend most of our waking time. We're hunched over, our shoulders slumped, our feet dragging. We're a generation who has sleepy glute muscles and flat butts.

The reason our glutes have gone to sleep is because of our modern living environment. Our lifestyles have done this to us. The way we live modern life is literally a pain in the ass. And this matters. We usually think of our bottoms as something to sit on, but they're actually one of the most important muscles in the body. They're a 'keystone' muscle and, if they're off, there can be knock-on effects for many other muscles. A lot of back pain is actually caused by having sleepy backsides. Glutes – our buttock muscles – not only help hold our skeletons up, they play a critical role in the functioning of our biomechanics. It's not by accident that men and women tend to, consciously or unconsciously, judge the quality of a potential mate partly on the shape of their butt. And our glutes do not exist in isolation. In our massively connected bodies, they're linked to a whole chain of muscles from our shoulders all the way down to our feet, and if they're not firing appropriately, that puts stress on other parts of the body.

I know first-hand how important these muscles are. When I was twenty-three I was a final-year medical student at Edinburgh University. I was moving into a new apartment for the year with my friends Steve and Mary. I was helping Mary move boxes up six flights of stairs with the most appalling posture you've ever seen. After about thirty minutes, I lifted a new set of boxes and boom! Sharp pain in my lower right back. I dropped all the boxes and fell to the ground in agony. My back had gone. Up until that point, I'd never given my back any thought. Like most of us, I abused it every day, as I'd never been given any reason not to. This led to ten years of chronic back pain which impacted all aspects of my life. I had to take time off work, carefully plan travel and give up all the sports that I loved.

I spent hours, not to mention thousands of pounds, seeking a solution. Everyone told me that, because of my height (I'm six foot six), back pain was inevitable. I simply refused to accept this and tried what felt like every therapy known to man. Most of them would give me short-term relief but within weeks the pain would come back. My desire to learn more led to me signing up to learn about movement mechanics with one of the subject's most revolutionary thinkers, Gary Ward. Gary is an incredibly important figure in the world of body mechanics and human movement. He's flipping all the old rules on their head and having great success in helping people. The brilliance of Gary's philosophy is that he's managed to simplify the huge complexity of the body's mechanics. Using his perspective, we can now work with the idea that the body's movements can be separated and worked with in just two primary chains.

FLEXOR CHAIN MUSCLES

The first one is the flexor chain. When we're curling our biceps or bringing our knees up to our chests, we're flexing. In our modern environment we tend to overuse our flexor chain. We're flexing our spines from the minute we get up to the minute we go to bed. We gawp at our smartphones with a flexed neck. A human head weighs between four and five kilograms, which is a big load to put on our neck joints each time we do this. We sit down to eat breakfast, sit down to get to work, hunch over a desk all day and then come home to sit on a sofa. This takes its toll. One of the main problems with sitting so much is that we're not giving our bodies the chance to experience the opposite posture. Things are so bad for many of us that we actually remain in this hunched, flexed state even when we do stand up! Clues that we are overusing our flexor chain include:

- Flat feet
- Knock knees
- Rounded upper back

- Forward head posture
- Sleepy glutes

EXTENSOR CHAIN MUSCLES

The opposite of the flexor chain is the extensor chain. We're using our extensor chain when our hips or spine are extended and upright. The muscles of extension enable us to stand up tall with our eyes on the horizon – the very opposite, in fact, of bad posture. The role of the extensor chain is to activate and pull us out of our flexed states. The key to achieving balance in our posture is to have full access to them both, so that the brain can choose what is optimal for the body's environment.

When the body's flexor and extensor chains are working together in balance, you see the classic 'book on head' posture:

- Standing up tall
- Long neck
- Head back

- Shoulders back and down
- Ribcage raised and elevated
- Glutes firing, active and switched on

Consciously trying to make these changes is not usually a successful long-term strategy. I spent years trying to implement the old commandment of pulling the shoulders back and standing up straight but it didn't work because I was not re-educating my brain. Gary's approach is aimed at moving the body to wake these extensor chain muscles up, switch your glutes on and make you stand up tall without even having to think about it.

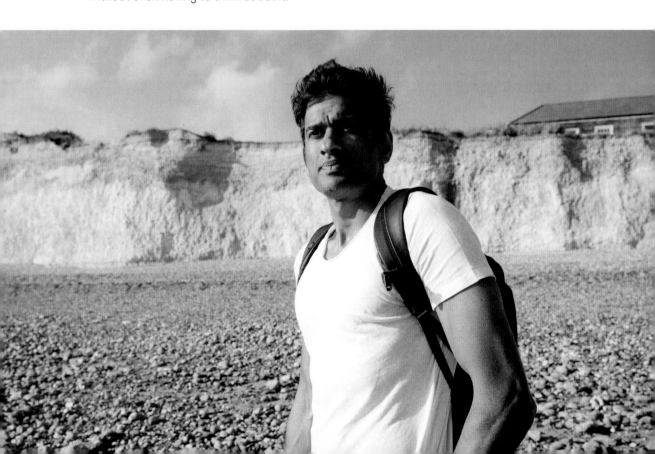

Because we spend so much of our modern lives hunched over, we've lost the ability to extend and be upright. We've got this almost foetal-like flexed posture from sitting in chairs and looking at screens and phones all day. A lot of the corrective work that people find themselves having to undergo involves restoring their powers of extension. When we fail to access our own extensor chain, one of the major muscle groups that deactivates and goes to sleep is the glutes.

EXTEND, EXTEND, EXTEND

This has been my mantra for the past few years and I hope it will become yours as well! We need to re-teach our body to extend. People struggle to extend their hips, people struggle to extend their spines. Of course, sitting less is extremely helpful but it doesn't automatically allow our bodies to experience extension. Most of us will need help in order to access our body's powers of extension in full.

When people are working on their bodies today, they tend to focus too much on the 'mirror muscles', which are the ones you can see in the mirror and so, naturally, the ones they prefer to work on. They get caught up in exercises that make the mirror muscles look good, such as bench presses, biceps curls and sit-ups. All these exercises ask the body to flex. We need far more focus on the muscles we can't see in the mirror, such as the ones on our back that extend the body and make it stand up straight.

As a teenager, a classic tall, skinny Indian kid, I remember being in the changing room at school and I could see my ribs. That made me extremely self-conscious. Meanwhile, I was being exposed to pictures of buff men in all the fitness magazines.

I started doing chest presses and sit-ups every day. I kept this up for about two years and, yes, I put on muscle. But I also inadvertently changed all of my body movement mechanics. Was it worth it? Absolutely not. I had to spend years in pain and then years of corrective exercising to undo the damage I'd caused. My mistake was being motivated purely by vanity and focusing on the mirror muscles. I see this whenever I'm in a gym – bodybuilders with overflexed and hunched shoulders, flat feet and rounded spines clearly walking around with poor posture and limited mobility.

I've always prided myself on being particularly open minded as a doctor and I'm always enthusiastic about learning about new things from different healthcare professionals. I was actually the first medical doctor to study with Gary, and what blew my mind about him was the fact that he saw the body in exactly the same way that I saw health. He was motivated by a desire to understand the root cause of problems, rather than simply suppress bodily symptoms. When I came to him with my back problem he very quickly identified that my right foot was 'stuck' in pronation. In other words, my foot arch had effectively collapsed and my foot was flat and so unable to access its opposite posture. Podiatrists had told me about my flat foot before but simply prescribed orthotic insoles, which hadn't worked.

Gary had a different solution. He told me he needed to get my right foot working again, insisting that was the key to my back problems. But, you might be thinking, what has this got to do with glutes? Well, in our massively connected bodies, there's actually a strong link between our foot muscles and our glute muscles. If one of our feet isn't working properly, this can directly affect our glutes, and vice versa. It turned out that my right glute muscle wasn't switching on and this meant my back was always going to struggle. My back was taking the strain instead of my sleepy backside.

Under Gary's guidance, it soon became clear why none of those, from physiotherapists to masseurs, who'd been manipulating my back over the years had solved the problem. They'd only ever been offering a temporary sticking-plaster fix. To completely heal my back, Gary had to teach me to reprogramme these damaging patterns and re-educate my body. I had to get my feet working correctly again. This, in turn, would reawaken my glute muscles. Incredibly, with just five minutes of exercise per day, over the course of less than a week, my longstanding back problems vanished. My exercises were based largely on the four I have detailed at the end of this section. It was the nearest thing to a miracle I've ever witnessed. Now, a few years on, I have a natural right-foot arch, my right glute is firing appropriately and my back pain has never resurfaced.

Thanks to Gary, my body has returned to its natural state. I'm now back to playing squash and skiing down mogul fields with no concerns at all. This has been completely life-changing for me. Day to day, I'm able to move my body more freely, re-engage with activities that I love but had to previously shun. This has had tremendous knock-on effects. I'm happier, fitter, have more energy and an improved sense of well-being. I'm living a life that was completely unimaginable to me only six years ago.

It was in Gary's brilliant book *What the Foot?* and on his training courses that I first learned about the importance of glutes, and how we must reawaken them in order to combat the effects of our flexed, hunched-over lifestyles. The glutes are extensor chain muscles. They aid the extension of the hip, which is the motion we make when standing up or coming out of a squat (as opposed to the flexion we make when bending at the hip to sit down). Hip extension and glute contraction should happen together. But in our super-flexed world, we're missing the ability to extend our hips properly. I want you to learn how to move your whole body to access hip extension using the following four exercises. I believe that these exercises will give your body the opportunity to awaken your glutes for evermore.

Some of you might have been through the rigmarole of extending your hips after many a physio session and you might even have come to the conclusion that it doesn't work. If so, I suspect, your discomforts have continued. But this is where Gary's unique philosophy kicks in. He believes that we've become flexed to such an extent that when we even try to extend, using the traditional exercises, we slip into bad habits. Our bodies have simply forgotten how to move as they should. Whenever we stand up, we're supposed to be using our glutes. Most of us don't. Our brains bypass the glutes, using other muscles. In order to retrain the brain, Gary has created a series of exercises that invite it to fire the right muscles. The important thing to know is that we can't simply consciously 'decide' to use our glutes and therefore extend properly. Our brains make these decisions for us, unconsciously. Therefore, we need exercises that remind the brain how to trigger the correct muscles. And this is exactly what Gary has designed.

Here's just one example. By bending the hip fully, we create a situation in which the only movement left available is one of proper extension. When we lie on our front and lift one of our legs, we should be doing it using our glute. But when instructed to do this, the brain has many options. Because our glutes are switched off, it tends to choose easier ones. Gary's movements make it so the brain has no option but to lift the leg in the proper way, using the glute.

Gary and I have come up with four movements that are designed to get your feet moving, your hips moving and your glutes working. They'll help retrain your brain to operate your body in accordance with the way it was designed. They can be carried out individually or as part of a group.

NB All movements should be made either barefoot or with socks on.

MOVEMENT ONE: FLEX ON A STEP

This can be any exercise step like a standard aerobics step, a baby step or even your lowest stair. The exercise is designed to wake up your glutes by flexing your hip joint. The step raises the foot off the ground, which encourages your hip flexion. As you bend and reach forward with your arms, you'll experience the glute lengthening. As you get to your end range of motion, which is the furthest point you can comfortably go, you'll naturally find yourself rocking back to the start position. You then go again. These movements are not to be held, like a stretch or a yoga pose. The idea is to gently move in and out of them, gradually increasing the range as you go.

1. Place one foot on a step and the other (the trailing foot) on the ground behind you, as in a stride.

2. Bend the knee of the front leg forward towards the toes. Avoid consciously controlling the movement of the knee, allow it to go where it comfortably wants to go, as you execute the movement. (Although the usual advice is to position the knee over the toe, Gary taught me that this actually limits our motion. Allowing it to follow the movements of the foot and hip is much more liberating for the body.)

3. As you bend the front knee, your hip will be drawn forward over the step towards the foot.

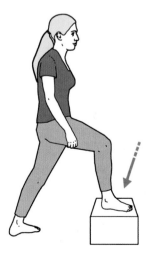 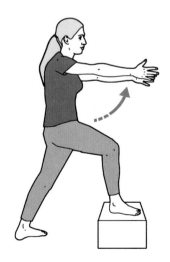

4. Gently reach out in front of you towards the horizon with your hands at hip height. As you move forward, the heel of the trailing foot will start to lift. This is perfectly normal.

5. As your hands reach forward at hip height, allow your upper body to follow as you attempt to reach as far as you comfortably can along this axis. (Your body should bend forward as a result of your hands reaching out.)

6. Our aim is to put most of our weight through the front foot on the step, with our hips sitting above the foot, and reaching forward with our arms, as in the picture.

7. As you become comfortable with this movement, and perhaps begin to find it easy, you can gradually lower your reach to knee height and out towards the horizon.

8. A long-term goal might be to safely place your fingertips on (or, ideally, beyond) the step. Do not hold these end positions but mindfully travel in and out of them back to upright.

9. Go as comfortably low as you feel is appropriate for you.

10. Repeat on the other leg.

For variation: reach forward with only either the right or left hand to this position.

For progressions of this movement, please see the online videos at drchatterjee.com

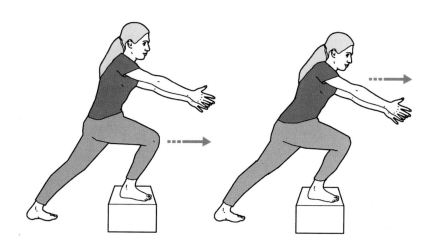

MOVEMENT TWO: THE HIP ADDUCTION

This movement wakes the glute up in more than one way. It uses flexion, but it also uses the lateral motion of the hip. This is a whole body movement which targets the glutes and many other muscles which constitute the extensor chain.

1. Stand on a step.

2. Choose a leg to stand on.

3. Whilst bending the knee of the standing leg, reach with the opposite foot behind and to the side, a bit like a curtsey, so that the toes of the reaching leg touch the floor.

4. Allow the weight-bearing knee to bend and to comfortably go where it wants. (Avoid consciously controlling the position of the knee.)

5. This begins to pull down the pelvis on the reaching-leg side and hike up the pelvis on the standing-leg side.

6. Raise the arm on the same side as your reaching leg and extend it towards the ceiling. When you reach high into your most comfortable end range, notice the stretch in that side of your abdomen.

7. You must maintain full weight bearing at all times on the standing leg. There is a temptation to put some weight on the reaching foot when it touches the floor. This should not happen – it should only tap the floor, not rest on it.

8. At your lowest comfortable point, bring yourself back up to standing and lower the opposite arm.

9. Allow both feet to rest on the step between repetitions of the same movement.

10. Change legs and repeat.

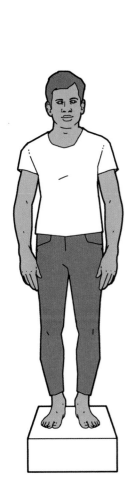
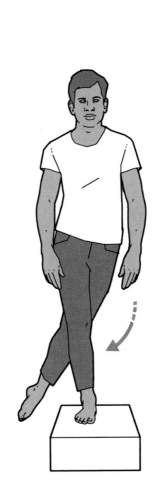
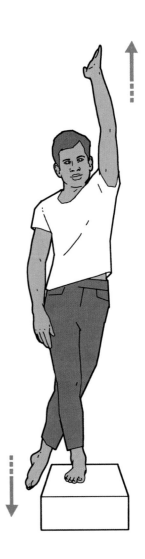

MOVEMENT THREE: FOOT CLOCKS

Your glute movements are connected to the movement of your feet. Healthy foot motion naturally contributes to the glute lengthening in the correct way. This exercise will help make this happen. In addition you can start to identify 'dark spaces' in your movement. These are the movements that your brain is not used to making. It's only by moving into these spaces that you can begin to reawaken pathways in your brain that have gone to sleep.

1. Start by standing with both feet together. Imagine yourself in the centre of a large clock.

2. Relax the toes and choose a leg to stand on.

3. With the toes of the other leg, tap lightly at clock position 12 o'clock. Keep the tapping leg straight whilst allowing the standing leg to bend. This should be as far as you can comfortably reach.

4. **Tap and return to the start position.**

5. **Most of your weight should remain on the standing leg. This is the one that remains in the middle of the clock-face.**

6. Allow the foot and knee of the standing leg to move freely as in the first two movements on the previous pages.

7. Begin a series of movements in which your reaching leg moves around the side of the clock that's the same side as your reaching leg (so, if standing on your right leg, follow the clock round from 12 anticlockwise to the left). Each time, ensure that the toes of the reaching leg only tap the floor lightly. The majority of your weight should remain taken by your standing leg.

8. Standing on your right leg aim to get as far round as 7 with the left leg (12,11,10,9,8,7). Then return to the start position before reaching to the next number on the clock face. Repeat this sequence between five and ten times.

9. Standing on your left leg aim to get as far round as 5 with the right leg (12,1,2,3,4,5).Then go back to the beginning. Repeat this sequence between five and ten times.

10. As the knee of your standing leg bends, and your other foot moves, your glutes will be encouraged to work.

11. Your focus is on the standing leg as the muscles react to the knee bending, the hip flexing and the foot flattening. The further your reach, the more you will be activating your glutes.

12. Ensure that you work both legs.

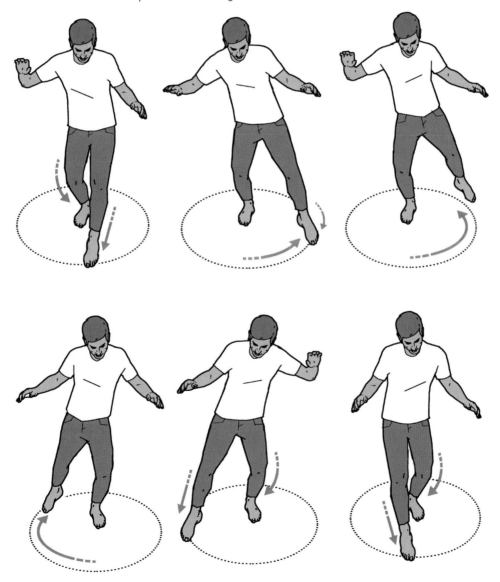

MOVEMENT FOUR: 3D HIP EXTENSION

This movement puts all the joints in the body into a position that gives the glutes no option but to be fully activated. The front leg will experience the lengthening of its corresponding glute whilst the back leg will experience a full glute shortening. Working both sides means you'll be able to experience the full range of motion for both glutes.

1. Start by standing with your feet hip-width apart.

2. Place one foot forward at a comfortable distance. This distance will vary between individuals and you will need to do some experimentation. Start with a distance of 50cm between the back foot big toe and the front foot one.

3. Relax the toes.

4. Bend the knee of your front foot whilst allowing the heel of the back foot to come up off the floor. You should keep the toes of the back foot on the ground.

5. Your weight should be mostly on the front foot. Try to let your pelvis move forward and come over your front foot.

6. Your torso should remain upright.

7. Try to think about your body moving forward and not down. This is not a gym-type lunge.

8. Keep the back knee straight and gently rotate it outwards, without bending it, whilst keeping the back toes pointing straight forward.

9. The idea is to keep your head over your ribcage, your ribcage over your pelvis, and your pelvis over your front foot – so you're all nice and stacked. If you feel any pressure in your lower back it's likely you're not achieving this.

10. Raise both arms towards the ceiling.

11. Return to the starting position. Do this between five and ten times on each leg.

12. When you become comfortable with this movement, try one of the multiple progressions shown at drchatterjee.com

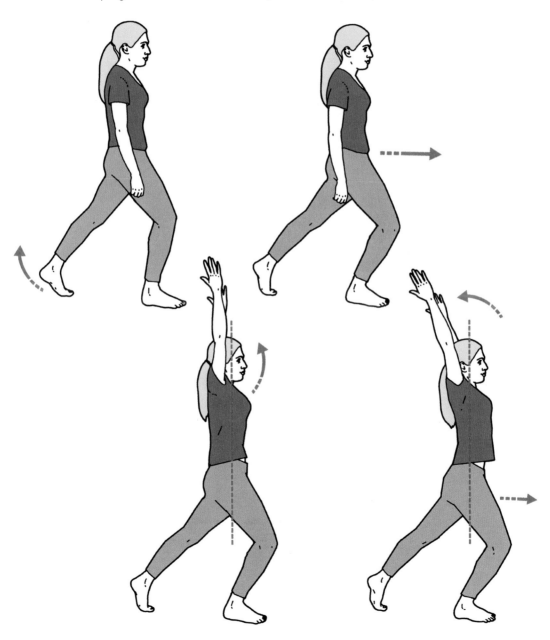

TIPS TO WAKE UP YOUR GLUTES

My recommendation is that you do *at least* one of these four movements every single day. Once you know what you're doing, they don't take long. Any one of them can take under a minute. What's more, these are not gym-style exercises that will get you all sweaty. You don't need to change clothes, you don't need to schedule them in, they won't make you lose your breath. It's crucially important to keep reminding your body that it should be switching your glutes on and the best part is, it takes hardly any time or effort at all.

I do these exercises every single morning, whilst my coffee's brewing, in order to prepare my body for the day ahead. If you can fit in all four of them in a quick five-minute morning movement session, all of your subsequent movements throughout the day will be more efficient and more in harmony with the way your body is designed to move. Try to do the whole series at least four times per week.

Note: If you have any concerns whatsover about performing any of the suggested movements in this pillar, you should consult a healthcare professional beforehand.

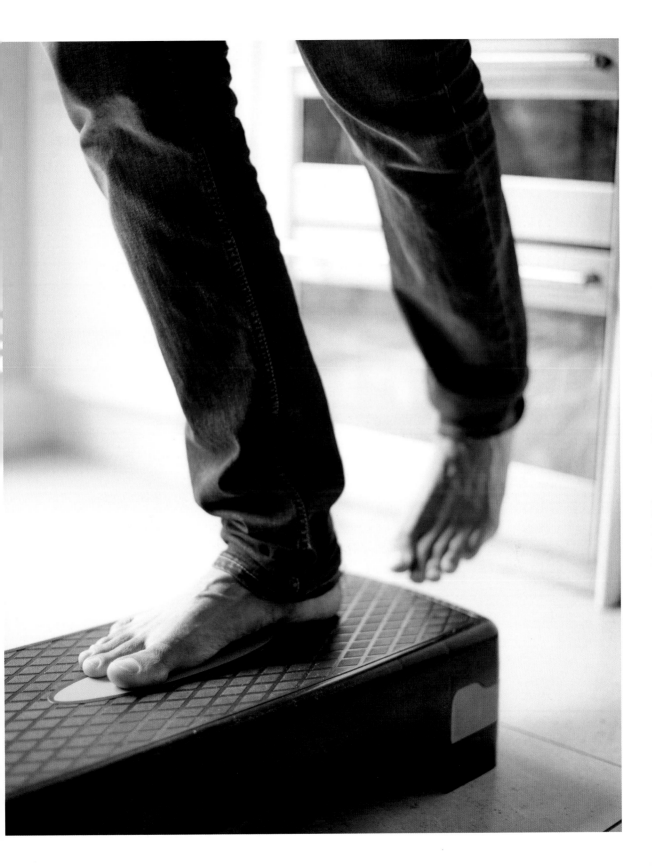

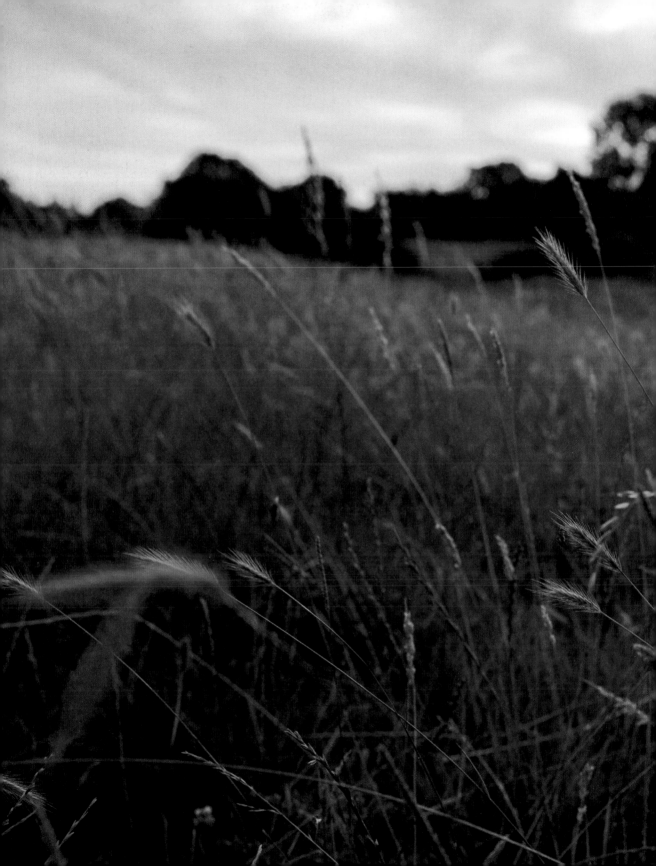

SLEEP

We're in the middle of a sleep deprivation epidemic. We not only have far too many distractions in our daily lives but we also live in a 'sleep is for wimps' culture that associates this natural and critical bodily function with laziness. Scientists from Oxford University claim we're getting between one and two hours less sleep per night than we did sixty years ago. In the context of an eight-hour sleep cycle, that's a hugely significant drop of up to 25 per cent. Want to know how damaging this is? It's actually possible to put a number on at least one aspect of it. Sleep deprivation is thought to cost the British economy about £40bn a year.

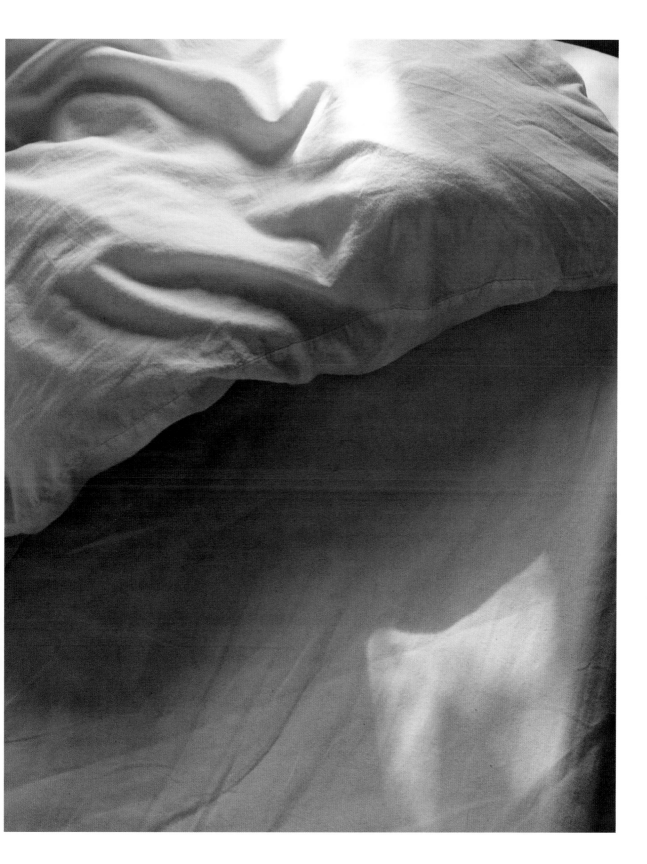

But this is a problem that goes far beyond financial cost. It's actively dangerous. Every time we drive when we're sleep deprived we're putting lives at risk. Recently I spent some time at a specialist centre in Guildford to see this for myself. Using a simulator, the test subject drove the same route three times – first under normal conditions, then after drinking enough alcohol to remain just under the drink-drive limit, and finally when he had been restricted to having only three hours sleep. When tired following his sleep restriction, he took up to four seconds to react to a hazard! This was a far worse result than when he'd had a drink. What I saw that day backs up a classic study from 1997 from the Queen Elizabeth Hospital in South Australia. The authors concluded that 'relatively moderate levels of fatigue impair performance to an extent equivalent to or greater than is currently acceptable for alcohol intoxication'. Whilst this in itself is extremely worrying, what sleep researchers find particularly dangerous is that many sleep-deprived individuals don't even realize they're fatigued, and their performance impaired. Their perception is that they're doing very well.

But who isn't guilty of cutting corners on their sleep? I see it all the time with my patients and I've done it myself. When I'm feeling tired on the sofa in the evening, it's so tempting to keep watching television, or mindlessly surf the internet rather than making an active decision to fall asleep. You know the score . . . and so do I. But as I've immersed myself in sleep research over the past few years, I've changed the priority I give to sleep. It's no exaggeration to describe the results as life-changing. I feel happier, stronger and more alert, and my productivity has improved significantly.

The legendary sleep researcher Dr Allan Rechtschaffen once wrote,

'If sleep does not serve an absolutely vital function, then it is the biggest mistake the evolutionary process ever made.'

I love that quote because it really captures something not only about the vastness of sleep but also of its mystery. Scientists are still teasing out some highly significant aspects of exactly what happens when we sleep, and there's still much we don't know. All animals sleep, and the consequences of not doing so can be drastic. Rats deprived of their shut-eye die within a month. The longest any human has managed to stay awake is a mere eleven days. When seriously sleep deprived, people usually hallucinate and can even have fits. The fact that we spend a third of our entire lives asleep just hints at how critical it is for both our mental and physical well-being. Getting sufficient high-quality sleep is essential for the proper functioning of our minds and bodies. It's a core physiological process that many of us inadvertently regard as optional. Professor Matt Walker at the University of Berkeley, California, says, 'There is no tissue within the body and no process within the brain that is not enhanced by sleep, or demonstrably impaired when you don't get enough.'

Here are just a few of the benefits we get from safeguarding our quality sleep time. During sleep, we allow the body to actively recover itself. As we discovered earlier (see page 108), the bodily spring-cleaning process known as autophagy is critical, and it's principally during sleep that our bodies mop up a lot of the waste that's accumulated in our cells during the day. It's thought that, when we sleep, our brain cells shrink in size to allow gaps to open up between our nerve cells, which allows our brain to wash away waste products that build up and accumulate whilst awake. To give one example, researchers believe that sleep is the time when we clear out the protein beta-amyloid, which accumulates in the brains of Alzheimer's patients. Sleep also helps us lay down new memories by promoting the growth of new nerve cells.

All three of the previous pillars feed directly into this one, and vice versa. When you sleep well, it's much easier to make better choices the following day. You crave less sugary food and feel more energetic, which, in turn, means you're inclined to be more physically active on the one hand and to engage in relaxation practices such as meditation on the other. Such behaviour is self-reinforcing: when you're more physically active, eat healthy food and prioritize relaxation, you'll sleep even better.

THE POTENTIAL BENEFITS OF A GOOD NIGHT'S SLEEP INCLUDE:

Increased energy

Improved concentration

Greater capacity to learn

Better ability to make healthy food choices

Improved immune system function

Enhanced autophagy

Reduced risk of developing chronic disease
such as type 2 diabetes

Better memory

Increased life expectancy

Reduced risk of being overweight

Reduced stress levels

Reduced risk of developing Alzheimer's

THE CONSEQUENCES OF NOT SLEEPING

I believe that sleep is arguably the most undervalued component of health in today's society. It has come to be regarded as optional, something we can do without. We're even made to feel as if we're somehow weak if we demand more and better sleep. But if we don't sleep, the consequences for our health can be serious. It's simply not true that we can get by perfectly well on insufficient sleep. It's a myth perpetuated by our modern culture and economy which values those who do more.

The damage it can do is widespread and serious. It is well recognized now that even short-term sleep deprivation causes increased levels of the stress hormone cortisol, raises blood pressure and impairs our body's ability to regulate blood sugar. It also activates our sympathetic nervous system, which can make us feel jumpy and stressed, increases levels of inflammation and decreases levels of leptin – the hormone that helps us feel full after eating. And there's a double hit in this respect, because it's been established that, when we're sleep deprived, we produce more of a hormone called ghrelin. Ghrelin stimulates hunger. So by not sleeping we feel less full thanks to one hormone and more hungry thanks to another. Now it should be starting to become clear why so many of us struggle to stick with our healthy food choices and exercise regimes. It also helps to explain why, if you sleep better, your goals for the other pillars will become much easier to achieve.

Plenty of studies link lack of sleep to obesity and type 2 diabetes. One found that just four nights' sleep deprivation caused significant insulin resistance whilst another argued that sleep problems may precede conditions such as anxiety and depression. Sleep also plays a role in our metabolic pathways, which affect how we manage blood sugar, and our immune system, which impacts how frequently we get a cold, how inflamed we are and even how our neural pathways work. The prestigious journal *Nature* published a revealing study in 2016 showing that long-term broken sleep in mice resulted in the following reversible changes:

- increased leptin levels (see page 134)

- increased gut permeability (leaky gut)

- increased inflammation

- increased fat mass

- increased insulin resistance

Similar mechanisms are thought to exist in the human body.

SLEEP DEBT

Unfortunately, we can't dodge the effects of sleep deprivation by having a bit of a lie-in on a Sunday morning. Studies show that we accrue 'sleep debt' which we can't just repay with a couple of cheeky extra hours here and there. One in particular looked at typical performance impairments that are caused by mild chronic sleep deprivation – which is the type that many of us are experiencing these days. It found that, even after three days of recovery, many of the debilitating effects remained. The consequences of sleep deprivation include:

- Increased risk of type 2 diabetes

- Increased risk of being overweight

- Decreased cognitive ability

- Poor performance at work

- Increased likelihood of being involved in a road traffic accident

- Increased chance of psychiatric disorders

HOW MUCH SLEEP DO WE NEED?

My definition of 'good sleep' is not a number. I don't know what the right amount of sleep is for you. It's not just a question of hours, it's also about quality. To assess the health of my patients' sleep I have devised a chart that I call 'RATE'. This involves three simple questions that provide an immediate snapshot of your sleep health.

- Waking up feeling **Refreshed** is a good general barometer of overall health.

- Waking up at the same time, give or take thirty minutes, without an **Alarm**, is a good indicator that your body's intrinsic biological rhythms are working well. (Some of you may find this question difficult because you have children or a pet that acts as your alarm – if so, just stick to the other two questions and score yourself out of 4.)

- Not being able to drop off within thirty minutes of trying (**Time Elapsed**) means that there is likely to be something in your lifestyle that is untraining your body's own natural ability to sleep.

A score of 0 indicates poor sleep health and a score of 6 is excellent. Anything under 6 means you could benefit significantly from the interventions in this pillar. Why not RATE your sleep now?

After scoring your own sleep and reading about the consequences of not getting enough, some of you may be starting to panic. There really is no need. In over sixteen years of practice I've learned that the majority of sleep problems are lifestyle related. This pillar is designed to help you identify what those lifestyle factors might be, and how you can actively change them.

How do you RATE your sleep?

Refreshed?	Alarm?	Time Elapsed?	Total
Do you wake up feeling refreshed?	Do you wake at the same time (within 30 minutes) every day without an alarm?	Do you fall asleep within 30 minutes?	

KEY

0– Never or rarely

1– Occasionally

2– Almost always

Many of my patients find that, most of the time, choosing three of the five interventions seems to be enough. Of course, all of the interventions will be helpful, but for many of us, doing all five will be unrealistic. I would love you to discover how many of them you need to do in the context of your life, in order to reach your own personal threshold. As you read through the Sleep pillar, start thinking about which interventions you can introduce into your life immediately. I have found that intervention 3, 'Create a bedtime routine', is particularly helpful. It focuses on actively winding down prior to hitting the sack and, hopefully, will soon have you sleeping like a baby.

1. CREATE AN ENVIRONMENT OF ABSOLUTE DARKNESS

Try to keep your bedroom completely dark and free of televisions or e-devices.

One of the simplest hacks I recommend is making sure the environment in which we go to bed is completely dark. Darkness is a signal to our bodies that it's time to rest. It triggers the production of melatonin, which is the hormone that's largely responsible for helping us go to sleep. People who enjoy camping will always tell you they sleep well. Why? Because they're suddenly immersed in the natural cycle of daily light that dims slowly, then they spend some time with perhaps a fire lit that gives out a particular kind of orangey yellow light. And then? Absolute darkness.

Over the past few years, I've become aware of the trend for hotel rooms to contain more and more light sources that don't switch off at night. Air conditioning controls, TV LEDs, electric alarm clocks, blue night-lights and much more besides. As technology advances, so the number increases. It can be hard to drop off with so many lights on. They feel intrusive to me and offensive. I've got into the habit of unplugging everything and even, when that can't be done, putting black tape over them. Some of my patients who frequently stay in hotels have also reported significant improvements in their sleep when they implement a no-tolerance policy for light. And what goes for hotel rooms also goes for our own homes, of course. Many of my patients have found that the glow of an electric clock can impact getting to sleep in the first place, or dropping back off if they wake during the night. Light pollution from street lamps is also very common. This is why I strongly recommend installing blackout blinds or extra-thick curtains.

To understand why controlling our bedroom light levels is so crucially important, we once again have to travel back many millennia, to the ancient eras in which the human machine was doing much of its evolving. All organisms on earth have evolved around the sun and humans are no exception. As we've already discovered, our bodies run on a complex symphony of cycles. Everything from our immune-system function, our gut function, our muscle strength and our hormones shows a daily rhythm. 'Circa' is Latin for 'around' and 'diem' (or 'dian') means 'day'. Controlling and conducting all of these circadian rhythms is the brain's master body-clock, the Suprachiasmatic Nucleus (SCN). All of our bodily functions are in some way influenced by the SCN. But the strange thing about it is that, without clues from the outside world, this clock system does not run precisely on a 24-hour cyle. What keeps our circadian clock system in time is light and dark cycles. It uses these clues from the outside world to make running adjustments to its timings.

This is why we're so sensitive to changes in light – and why messing with them can have such powerful effects. When we abuse our exposure to light, we abuse our body clock. We shift it forwards or backwards, which throws many of our cycles out of whack. And yet too little light in the morning and too much at night is increasingly the norm these days.

SUPRACHIASMATIC NUCLEUS (SCN)

- The SCN is the master regulator of our body's internal clock

- It sits in a part of our brain called the hypothalamus

- It orchestrates all of our body's functions by synchronizing and coordinating with all of our body's other clocks

---

Over at the Sleep and Circadian Neuroscience Institute at Oxford University, Professor Russell Foster is one of Britain's foremost researchers in this area. He's called us 'the supremely arrogant species' because we think we can override the millions of years of evolution that created these rhythms within us. I love that line. It's spot on. We think we can stay up late under artificial light without consequences for our health. We forget the extraordinary power light has over the human machine. Light is a drug. It changes parts of the body on a molecular level. It changes the way certain genes are expressed. And most of us have no idea just how sensitive we are to it.

One remarkable study suggested that, even when our eyes are closed and a torch is shone behind our knees, our circadian rhythm can be affected. Although some scientists have argued about that study's reproducibility and its exact significance, it certainly supports the broader idea that there may be light-sensitive mechanisms that do not involve the eye. In any event, even if our eyes are firmly closed, light can still penetrate the eyelids.

EXPOSURE TO BRIGHT LIGHT

Exposure to bright light after sunset is a modern phenomenon. It began with the advent of street lighting about a hundred years ago, but in the past decade the problem has become a great deal worse with the boom in electronic devices, and the habit so many of us have got into of taking them to bed with us. Of course, some exposure to artificial light is essential. We can no longer simply choose to go to sleep when it gets dark. What we can do, though, is try to limit the effects of our modern light-filled lifestyles.

SMARTPHONES AND TABLETS

One of the worst things you can do in the hour or two before bed is look at your smartphone or tablet. Believe it or not, these electronic devices emit the same wavelength of light as the morning sun. Confusingly, it's called 'blue light', and just by looking at our phones, we're duping our bodies into thinking it's the start of the day. You're giving your brain a signal that says, it's not bedtime. When that blue light hits the back of your retinas, signals are sent to your pineal gland telling it not to make any more of the sleep hormone melatonin. We know that even a glance at the light a smartphone emits can impact melatonin secretion.

In order to mitigate this, I've installed an application called f.lux on my iPhone that lowers the amount of blue light emitted from its screen. Versions are also available for Mac, Windows and Android operating systems. There is also an app called Twilight for Android phones. Apple and many Android phones now come with their own night-time mode that alters both the intensity and the frequency of the light your phone emits, enabling you to reduce blue light emissions without the use of an app. This isn't as good as going without your phone completely, but it is a step in the right direction for those of us who are inseparably attached to our devices. If you really must look at them late at night, I'd recommend buying some amber glasses. The amber lenses help to filter the blue light from your screen. I have patients who can feel extremely sleepy within an hour of wearing them, which tells me how great an effect blue-light exposure had been having. Amber glasses usually work better than the apps, and can be bought online for as little as £10.

At home, my wife and I have tried to institute a rule that says unless there's some kind of exceptional circumstance, our phones and laptops go off at 8.30 and we don't bring them upstairs. I know that if I bring my phone upstairs, almost without realizing what I'm doing, I'll find myself scrolling down my social media feeds and the next thing I know I'm wide awake thinking about the news story I've just read or seeing the halo of light from the screen still flashing behind my eyes. Do we always manage to stick to this rule? If I'm being compeletely honest, the answer is no. But when we do, we both feel the difference.

TELEVISION

What goes for e-devices also goes for television. Many of us like to watch TV in the evenings. Unfortunately it's now well established that viewing time correlates with an increased risk of all-cause cardiovascular disease mortality. In short, it appears that the more television you watch, the more likely you are to die. Why? There are lots of theories about this, including that it's a sedentary pastime, but I can't help but wonder about the effect of all that bright light before bed. Is it messing with our circadian rhythms? One of the functions of light and the circadian clock is to signal to our bodies when it's time to eat. The good news is, when you restrict your eating times as described in the Eat pillar, you spontaneously reduce your calorie intake and you're also getting your food when your body is attuned and expecting to get it. What's more, assuming you're eating in daylight hours, restricting your food window also helps normalize your circadian rhythm, which aids sleep.

I recommend that you remove your television from your bedroom completely. If you must watch it in the evening, turn it off at least thirty minutes before going to bed. (I'd love you to push this to ninety minutes, but I do understand that this will be hard for many.) Although televisions do emit blue light, the fact that you're further from the screen makes it less of an issue than with tablets and smartphones. If you do end up in front of the TV in the evening, consider what you're watching. The news can be full of grief, trauma and anxiety – is that what you need inside your brain right before bed? Perhaps a feel-good film, a light-hearted comedy or a travel documentary would be more positive and calming?

EMBRACE RED LIGHT

So you now have a perfectly dark sleeping environment. Your e-devices have been expelled and your bedroom television is in the shed. You have blackout blinds installed, or extra-thick, well-fitted curtains. Light has been systematically abolished. But what happens if you need to get up in the night? In cases like these, or if your kids demand a night-light, you should consider using red light. Red is the wavelength that has the least impact on your body's circadian clock.

My own experience with this has been life changing. Like many of you, I have young children. They've always been early risers and I'm OK with that, as they go to bed pretty early. They've always liked having a night-light and we used to put a dim white one on in the corridor outside their room. However, after reading the research on red light, I bought one for their bedroom instead. This instantly caused them to sleep for an hour longer than they used to. I've heard similar stories in my surgery.

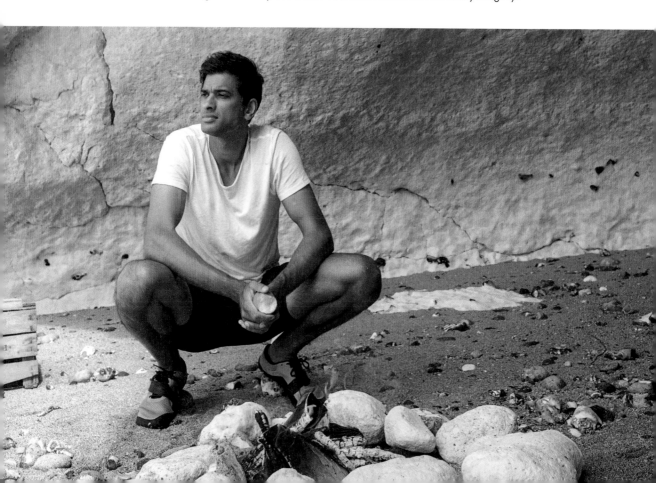

STARING AT THE SUN

I've had many patients for whom lighting adjustment was a game changer. Recently I saw Isabelle, a thirty-four-year-old who'd been struggling with fatigue. She didn't have any other health complaints, just a general lack of energy. Once we dug a little deeper into her life, it became clear that sleep had become an issue. She'd tried all kinds of things in the past including over-the-counter sleep aids and even stronger sleeping pills. As we chatted, I discovered that she spent the last ninety minutes before turning out the light staring at her phone. 'This is like staring at the sun right before closing your eyes for sleep,' I told her. 'You're giving your body a signal to be awake.' But as hard as I tried, I just couldn't convince her to go without her phone. We eventually compromised on a pair of amber glasses.

Instantly, she started to sleep better. A few weeks later she came back and was so convinced by what I'd told her that she actually started to switch off her devices ninety minutes before bed. She now puts on her amber glasses at 7.30 p.m. to block out all blue light in the evening. Once she gets to 9.30 p.m. all her screens go off. She then falls asleep at around 11 o'clock. And what difference has all this made to her? She's like a new person, and it's all because she sleeps better. She now makes healthier food choices, her mood is elevated and she exercises more.

Isabelle is a classic example of how making changes in one pillar feeds into all the other pillars. Once we did one thing that started to improve the way she felt, it triggered a cascade of benefits which, in turn, gave her the energy and motivation to make further improvement. She is living, breathing, thriving proof of the incredible power of making simple, sustainable changes to your lifestyle.

TIPS TO HELP YOU EMBRACE DARKNESS

FIT CORRECTLY SIZED EXTRA-THICK CURTAINS OR, EVEN BETTER, BLACKOUT BLINDS ✓

REMOVE ALL SCREENS FROM YOUR BEDROOM (LAPTOPS, PHONES, TELEVISIONS) ✓

BUY AN OLD-FASHIONED ALARM CLOCK ✓

ENSURE ANY LANDING CURTAINS ARE BLACKED-OUT AND DRAWN. LIGHT CAN EASILY LEAK INTO YOUR BEDROOM FROM ELSEWHERE IN THE HOUSE ✓

LEAVE YOUR CHARGERS IN ANOTHER ROOM TO AVOID BRINGING YOUR PHONE INTO THE BEDROOM ✓

BUY A RED NIGHT-LIGHT ✓

BUY AMBER GLASSES TO HELP MINIMIZE BLUE-LIGHT EXPOSURE IN THE EVENING ✓

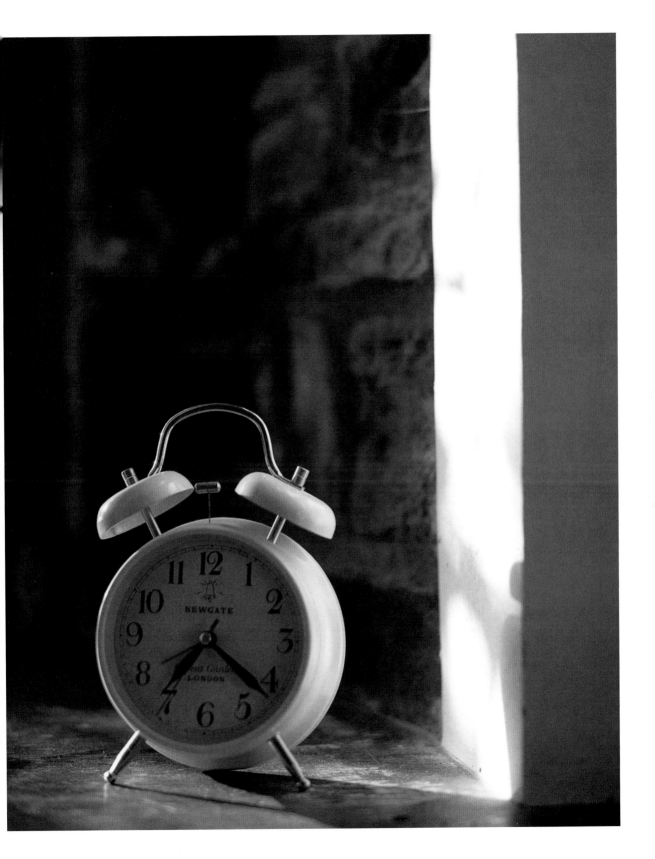

2. EMBRACE MORNING LIGHT

Spend at least twenty minutes outside (without sunglasses) every morning.

By making conscious changes to our lifestyle we make unconscious changes to our biology. At any given moment, untold numbers of complex and vital processes are starting, stopping and running in our bodies, and a great many of them rely on signals from the outside world to know when and how to run. We've just talked about how making the conscious decision to manage the darkness levels in our sleeping environments can trigger a wealth of unconscious processes that first help us get to sleep, then help us sleep better, and *then* have a number of amazing effects on our health and decision making. But, just as we should manage darkness at night, we should also manage our light in the mornings.

Prioritizing sleep starts the minute we get up and one of the best things we can do is get outdoors in natural daylight. Our exposure to the sun in the morning is a critical part of our evolutionary heritage. It's critical for feelings of well-being in the day but also for good quality sleep at night. Over the past two years, I've even found myself persuading some of my patients to have their morning cup of tea in the garden with a fleece on. (I'm still working on my mother; she's taken on board nearly all my lifestyle advice, but this one is proving to be a challenge for her.)

You might doubt the point of all this when you look out of your window and see it's a typically grim and dim British day. But it doesn't matter if it's cloudy. Even on the dullest days, we're still exposing ourselves to light at a higher amount outdoors than if we were in. Light is quantified in units called lux. Full sunlight gives us about 30,000 lux and going outside on a cloudy day gives roughly 10,000. If we're in a brightly lit indoor room, we're unlikely to be getting any more than 500 lux. What's more, the retinal photoreceptors that exist in the eye are most sensitive to a short wavelength blue-green light. In nature, we get exposure to this light only in the morning hours. This light information goes to our central body clock, or SCN, which, through the nervous system, orchestrates all of our body's peripheral clocks and rhythms.

The differential between your maximum and minimum light exposure is also important in helping set your body's rhythms. If you wake up and have breakfast at home indoors, travel to and from work in an enclosed vehicle and spend all day inside a building, you may hardly ever be outside. Your body is almost never exposed to natural light. You probably won't ever hit above 500 lux. Clearly, that has huge potential to disrupt your body's rhythms.

Getting the right kind of light at the right point in the day can have amazing effects throughout our bodies. Researchers in a 2014 study gave subjects a special wristwatch that also measured their exposure to light as well as their physical activity levels. It was found that the individuals who received more morning light had lower body mass indexes. Meanwhile, an observational study from 2016 followed the health habits of nearly 30,000 women. It found that smokers who had a high degree of sun exposure had the same risk of mortality as non-smokers who did not expose themselves to the sun. The lead author of that paper concluded that 'avoidance of the sun may be a risk factor for health in the same magnitude as being a smoker'. This is only an observational study, so it's hard to tease out causation at this stage, but I do believe these intriguing findings warrant further investigation, and certainly support our growing awareness of the sun's importance.

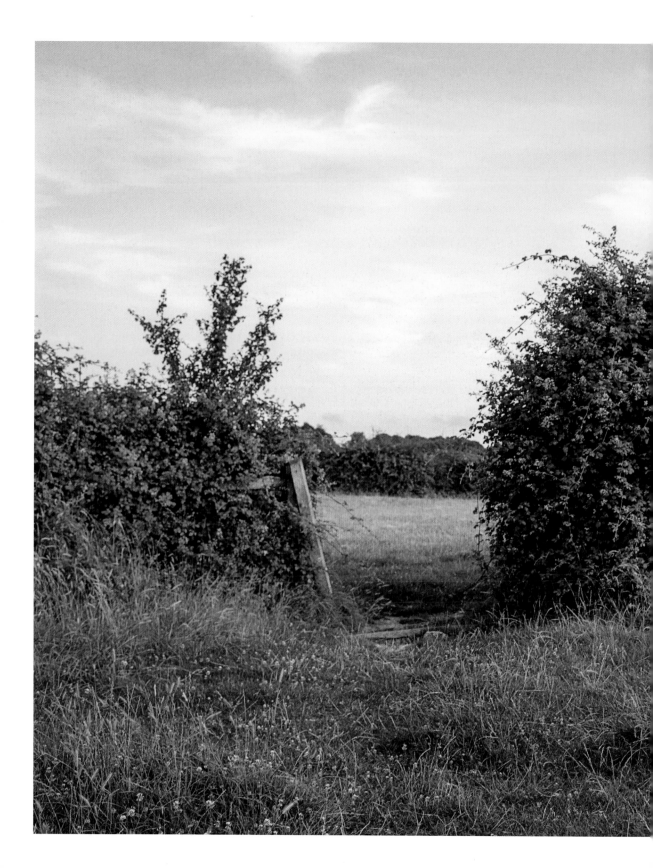

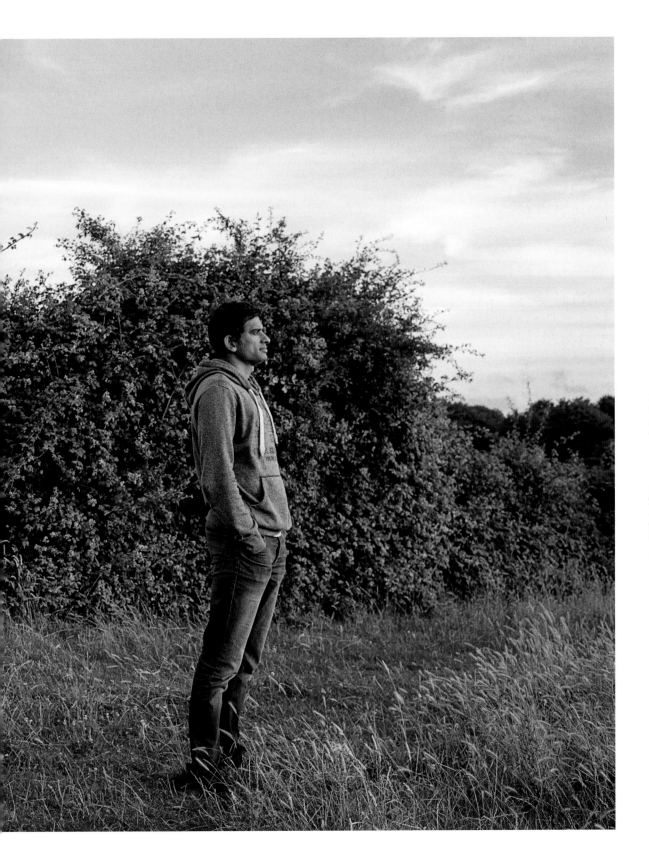

NATURE DEFICIENCY

An additional benefit to all this is that being outside for twenty minutes every morning means we're much more likely to be exposing ourselves to nature. I believe that as a society we're suffering from a nature deficit. It's now well established that doing activities in nature is associated with improved psychological well-being. It's also been established that the more urbanized our environment, the worse our health. There are many reasons for this, but the World Health Organization says that the urbanization of the planet is having a significantly negative impact on us. The fact is that working out in a soulless gym under artificial light is just not as good for you as working out in nature.

A study by researchers in Australia found that those who exercise outdoors on a regular basis have higher levels of serotonin, which is a hormone thought to be involved in happier moods. It also helps reduce fatigue. If you're working out outdoors you're much likelier to be able to exercise for longer, because you don't have that boredom and fatigue. Being in nature also helps you switch off. We can't always get to nature every day; either there's no park nearby or perhaps the time pressure involved makes it simply impossible. But most of us should, at the very least, be able to get outside. Even if we are waiting at a bus stop, for example, we can look at the trees, listen to the birds, get lost in a trance as we gaze at the branches moving in the wind.

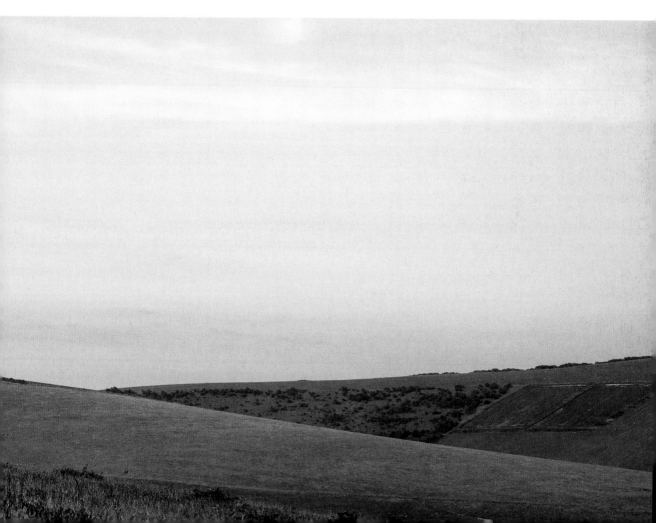

I know it sounds almost crazy, but I truly believe companies should start giving staff regular light breaks. One of the big problems with our approach to health is that we're preoccupied with sickness and disease rather than well-being. We prioritize reactive healthcare rather than proactive action. I am convinced that if employers took this seriously, they'd have enhanced productivity from their employees. Remember that mid-morning walking break that I take in my surgery?

Yes, it gives me a dose of much needed 'me' time and helps towards my 10,000 steps, but it also exposes me to natural light, clears my mind, makes me more efficient when I get back and helps me to sleep better at night. I'm hitting three of the four pillars with one change.

Another tip to get more natural light exposure is to avoid sunglasses in the morning. We want the natural sunlight (or even just daylight) getting into our eyes. That said, I also have many patients who work night shifts and it can be extremely useful for them to manipulate light using sunglasses. I often recommend to these patients that they use bright-light lamps at work during the night to help them stay awake but then to cut out light during the later part of the shift and wear sunglasses on the way home. I wish I'd known this ten years ago when I was a junior doctor and seemed to be constantly on night shifts. I always had difficulty sleeping in the day when on a run of seven nights. By the end of the week I'd be shattered. I'd also feel quite depressed. I often wonder how different things might have been if I'd applied the principles of circadian biology back then.

These days I make a habit of going into my garden every morning. Clearly, this is much more pleasant in the height of summer than the grim depths of winter, but even on the coldest days I'll put on a thick jacket and sit in the garden enjoying my coffee. I also try to go for a twenty-minute walk at some point during the morning.

I recently saw Barry, a retired bus driver who'd been struggling with his sleep for years. His was a puzzling case. He watched television with his wife every evening but always switched it off before 9.30. Then he would read in bed next to a dim light for approximately half an hour before settling down. Despite these good habits, since his retirement Barry's sleep quality had slowly been deteriorating. He was finding it harder to get to sleep and was waking up feeling unrefreshed. It turned out he was spending a lot of his day inside. Although his working life had been spent driving, the big windows of his bus exposed him to generous amounts of daylight. But now he was spending most of his time in his garage, tinkering with his beloved electric train set.

He was reluctant to do much, as his poor sleep was sapping his energy, but I managed to persuade him to go for a thirty-minute walk every morning. We identified a newsagent fifteen minutes away, where he'd go to get his daily paper. This ensured he was being exposed regularly to natural light. At my next two-week follow-up appointment, he reported that he was falling asleep faster and waking up more refreshed. In addition, he so enjoyed his morning walk that he started to go for an afternoon one every day as well, around a neighbouring park.

One of the great things about this intervention is that you can combine it with others. If you use this time outside as your daily workout, you're ticking off another box in the Movement pillar. It also helps with 'me' time from the Relax pillar, and you are more likely to reach your 10,000 steps a day. But whether you combine it with one of the other interventions or not, if you make light a priority, I promise you will very quickly start to feel the difference.

7 TIPS TO HELP YOU EMBRACE MORNING LIGHT

Pick two or three that work for you.

- HAVE YOUR MORNING TEA OR COFFEE IN THE GARDEN OR NEXT TO A WINDOW

- DON'T GET YOUR NEWSPAPER DELIVERED; COLLECT IT YOURSELF ON FOOT

- IF YOU MUST DRIVE IN THE MORNING, LEAVE THE CAR A TEN-MINUTE WALK AWAY FROM YOUR DESTINATION

- IF YOU SHOP IN THE MORNING, PARK AS FAR AS POSSIBLE FROM THE SUPERMARKET ENTRANCE

- GET OFF THE BUS HALF A MILE FROM YOUR DESTINATION AND WALK THE REMAINING DISTANCE

- CONSIDER GETTING A DOG AND TAKING IT FOR A WALK EVERY MORNING

- TRY TO TAKE A MORNING BREAK AND GO FOR A SHORT WALK OUTSIDE

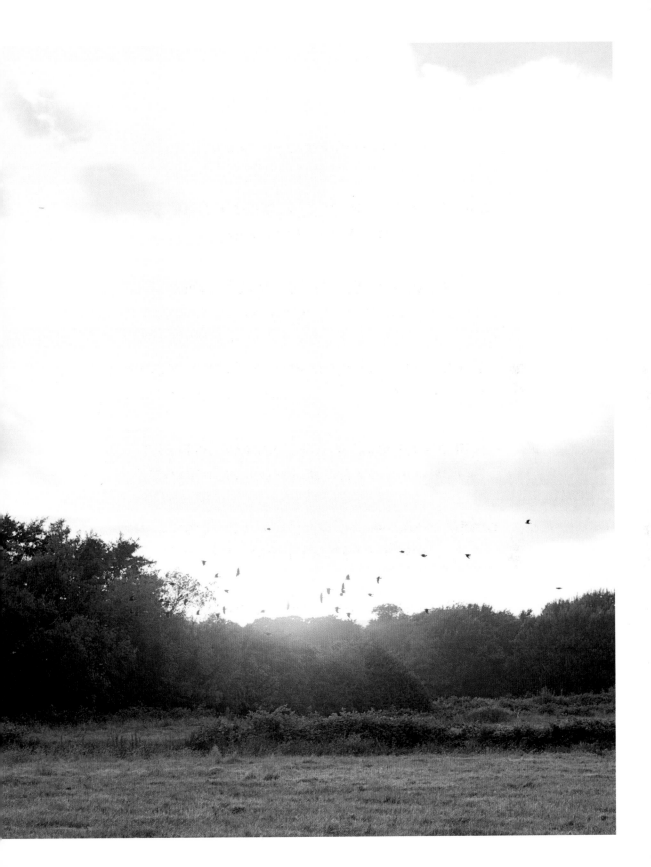

3. CREATE A BEDTIME ROUTINE

Start your evening wind-down with a 'No-Tech 90'
as part of a set ritual.

Contrary to popular belief, every single one of us has amazing natural rhythm. Whilst this might not always be obvious when we're busting moves down at the club on a Saturday night, our bodies do in fact run on an elegant, complex system of inner rhythms. As noted elsewhere, we all have a master body clock that keeps its time using signals of light and dark. But our liver also has its own rhythm. So does our blood pressure, our memory, our insulin, our production of the sleep hormone melatonin, our production of the hunger hormone leptin, our core body temperature, our mood, our memory, and so on. We now know that our genome is under much more clock control than we previously imagined, meaning that the very way our genes function can shift with time. It's now thought that a significant part of our genome may be clock dependent (which means there might be an optimum time when a liver drug, for example, would be most effectively administered). All these rhythms combine to form the awe-inspiring and beautiful symphony that is the healthy human body.

So the body has its own intrinsic rhythms and we need to try and support them. Aside from having a regular sleep time, one way we can do this is by having a constant routine or pathway that leads us towards sleep. This will help us not only to nod off more quickly, and enjoy richer sleep, but also to get out of bed feeling more refreshed. We've all got a daily or 'diurnal' variation in our cortisol (see page 23), which is a hormone that helps make us active and alert. It *should* help us bounce out of bed full of energy for the day. It usually peaks around one hour after waking, after which it embarks upon its slow and steady decline for the rest of the day. Breaking these routines can have all sorts of unpleasant consequences. Sleeping in at the weekend, for example, is a well-known trigger for migraine sufferers.

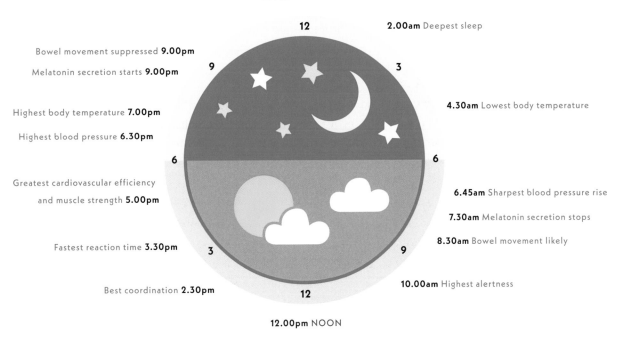

12.00am MIDNIGHT

2.00am Deepest sleep

Bowel movement suppressed **9.00pm**

Melatonin secretion starts **9.00pm**

Highest body temperature **7.00pm**

Highest blood pressure **6.30pm**

4.30am Lowest body temperature

Greatest cardiovascular efficiency
and muscle strength **5.00pm**

6.45am Sharpest blood pressure rise

7.30am Melatonin secretion stops

8.30am Bowel movement likely

Fastest reaction time **3.30pm**

10.00am Highest alertness

Best coordination **2.30pm**

12.00pm NOON

A study from June 2017 put these ideas to the test. Sixty-one university students were examined for thirty days using a special metric called the sleep regularity index. The researchers analysed the students' sleep patterns, the timing of their melatonin secretion and their academic performance. They found that irregular sleep schedules were associated with significant changes in circadian rhythms as well as poorer academic performance, concluding that the effect of keeping irregular sleep schedules was akin to jetlag, affecting us as much as travelling two to three zones westward.

Having said all that, I do know that sticking to the same bedtime constantly is not always going to be possible. The reality is that there will be times when you stay up later than is ideal, whether it's a friend's party, a dinner date, work engagements or whatever. In these situations, I make one simple recommendation. No matter how late you are to bed, no matter if the next day is a Monday or a Sunday, always get up at the same time. It's my experience that this is one of the most important things you can do for your health.

I know what you're thinking. Doesn't this completely fly in the face of what I've just told you, about the importance of getting enough sleep and avoiding fatigue? It does. Which is why I want you to embrace the habit of napping. Of course, you will have missed out on sleep, but for most of us, staying in sync is better than catching up in the morning. If you did stay up late the night before and are still feeling tired in the morning, it is worth trying to catch up with a microsleep.

ALARM FOR BEDTIME

Just as important as having a set getting-up time is having a fixed routine for going to bed. I remember reading about the superstar chef Jamie Oliver, and how he realized he hadn't been prioritizing his sleep for years. To prompt him, he started using a wearable tracker device that would literally buzz when it was time to go to bed. I really love this idea of having an alarm for bedtime. You should make your alarm a signal that the wind-down for bed must begin and set it for ninety minutes before lights out. And as soon as it sounds, that's when your No-Tech 90 begins. This is when you turn off all your e-devices, including computers. No exceptions. (I don't mind a bit of TV, but would really prefer this to go as well.) We're all aware that children need their own bedtime routine. We don't stimulate them at night, we wind them down: a relaxing bath followed by a bedtime story in dim light. It all helps to wind them down and create the correct environment and atmosphere for dropping off into deep, healthy, relaxing sleep. Why do we as adults feel that things should be any different?

MY IDEAL NIGHTIME ROUTINE

This is what I strive for although, with the pressures of work and family life, I only manage this a few nights per week. It is important that you find a routine that suits you and your lifestyle.

- I make sure that all my vigorous exercise is done by 6.30 p.m.

- By 8.30 my mobile phone and computer have been switched off (my No-Tech 90 starts here).

- A dim red light goes on in the hall (the kids like this as a night-light).

- Occasionally I'll watch a bit of TV, but if I do it'll be something relaxing, and I'll be doing some light stretching at the same time.

- Sometimes I sit and listen to relaxing music, or do some deep breathing in silence.

- If thirsty, I sip on non-caffeinated herbal tea or water.

- I head to bed around 9.30.

- I ensure the bedroom window is open a little. Many of us, with central heating, have our bedrooms too warm. Much better to have a cool bedroom and snuggle under a duvet.

- I read next to a dim light until I feel ready to fall asleep.

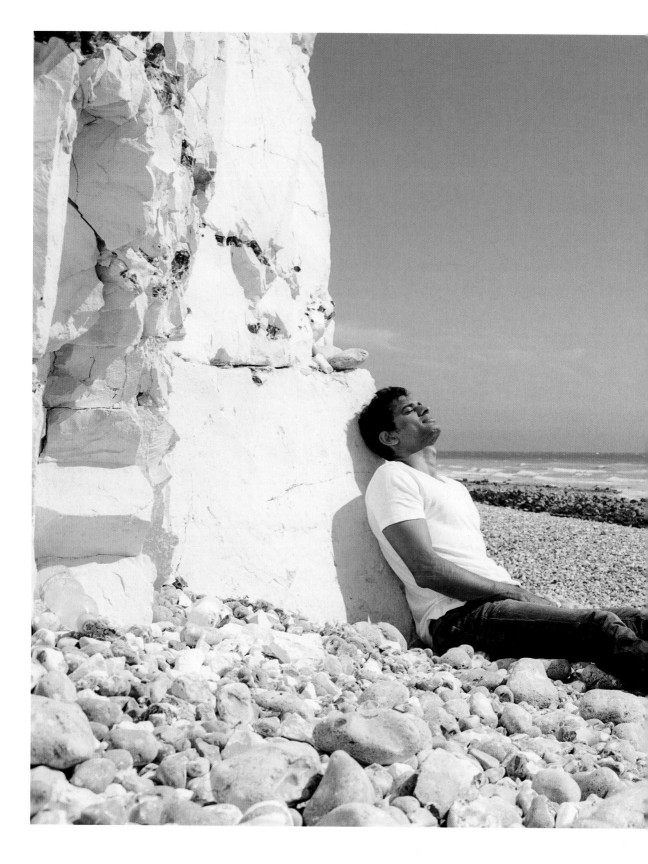

MICROSLEEPS

I define a microsleep as any time period in the day when you drop off, be it for five minutes at your desk all the way up to two hours in bed. I think we should embrace these microsleeps rather than worry that they will adversely affect our sleep at night.

I'm a huge fan of them, and they're associated with all kinds of benefits. On the Greek island of Ikaria, which is one of those quasi-magical 'blue zones' that are of huge interest to scientists because of their stunning rates of longevity, all the residents nap. Naps have been linked to a plethora of health benefits, including increased vigilance, improved ability to add numbers, alertness, reaction times and logical reasoning. The space agency NASA found that if co-pilots took a twenty-six-minute nap their alertness improved by 82 per cent. A study carried out by Professor Richard Wiseman for the Edinburgh International Science Festival suggested that short naps can even boost our happiness. Some of my patients grab naps in their car, whilst I've been known to lie on the examining couch for fifteen minutes. I have found it very useful for perking up my energy levels and focusing on afternoon surgery.

Of course, if you do feel your afternoon nap is adversely affecting your ability to sleep at night, it might be worth reducing the amount or stopping. In my experience though, most patients sleep better at night when napping in the day.

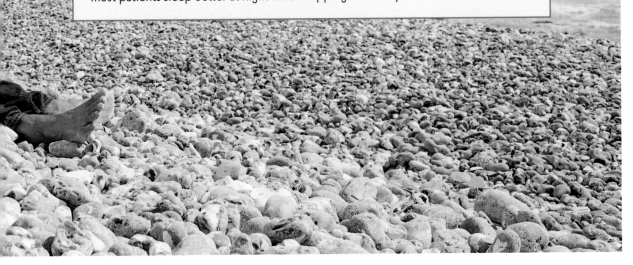

4. MANAGE YOUR COMMOTION

Minimize any activity that will raise emotional tension before bed.

This intervention is about reducing emotional tension or stimulation in the precious 'campfire hours' before bed. For the majority of sleep problems that I see, 'emotional commotion' in the last part of the day plays a big contributory role. (Emotional commotion is simply the term I use to describe being in a state of alert anxiety, or, in common parlance, 'a bit wound up'.)

Managing your commotion means making it a cast-iron rule that you do not discuss emotive subjects in the evenings, or crack into a new work task, or check your bank balance or do anything that's going to set your mind working. If you know watching *Question Time* is going to get you all het up then either avoid it altogether or watch it on a Saturday morning, when you've the time and the cortisol to deal with it. Of course, it's very hard to diarize an argument with your partner, but if you know you need to have a difficult conversation, don't have it at bedtime. It is probably wise not to watch thrillers, either. This might sound trivial but, remember, sleep deprivation is a major contributor to the epidemic of lifestyle diseases that we're currently in the grip of. It really is that important.

LEARN TO SAY NO

One of the ways I used to get this wrong was by being too much of a 'yes' man. I still try to be – and hope I am – a guy who does things for other people, but there was a period when I let other people's needs completely overwhelm my own. I didn't take ownership of my time. I was always thinking, 'Well, they want me to do that. What can I do? I can't say no.' But I've since learned to be a little selfish and to protect my own time. In our modern society, time is a precious commodity – more precious than gold, if you ask me. I've come to see taking someone's time as almost as serious a transgression as taking their money. People shouldn't feel entitled to our time, just as we shouldn't feel we have to give our cash to anyone who asks.

I've let the people around me know that after 8 p.m. I do not want to be contacted about anything that can wait until morning. Unless it's an emergency, I don't want to know about it. I have a lot of work contacts in the US and often they used to schedule calls for 9 or 10 p.m. Now they wait until the following day. If my wife wants to go through some deep stuff to do with the kids or the logistics of something I'll tell her, 'Babe, I don't want to do it now. I'm on wind-down.'

I see a lot of patients who find this hard. But if we're to manage our commotion successfully, the first thing we have to do is define our own boundaries and stick to them. In the past I thought it was rude not to reply to every email I received. Now I've changed my view. Before the age of email, did I reply to every item of post that came through my letterbox? Did I write to the manager of the local Domino's and thank her for her kind offer of a buy one, get one free? Of course I didn't. Let's say on a Friday night I've got thirty emails to go through, which isn't uncommon. I've got a choice. Do I abide by an agenda that other people have set for me? Or do I prioritize my own health, happiness and time with my family at the weekend? I make no apology for choosing the latter. I've taken back control.

One reason I don't respond to anything but emergencies after 8 p.m. these days is that I know a racing mind is one of the biggest causes of suboptimal sleep. In 2012 I came across a large UK sleep survey that really stuck with me. It revealed that the most common persistent thoughts that kept people up at night were as follows:

- Thinking about what they had done today and what they had to do tomorrow

- Thinking about how long they had been lying awake for

- Thinking about trivial things of no importance

- Thinking about what the future holds

- Thinking about things that happened in the past

The most common one, which was reported by an incredible 82 per cent of respondents, was the first – thinking about what they had done, and had to do. Sound familiar? We all know this feeling. This is one of the main reasons students struggle to sleep around exam time. Such thoughts are racing through their minds as they are lying in bed. This does not make for good sleep.

This intervention is really about the creation of new habits. It's about training people around you, about learning to say no and taking control of this part of your evening. Although I appreciate it's not always easy, it's also about drawing boundaries at work. Modern technology often blurs the line between where work stops and where our own lives begin. It's incredible to think that, thirty years ago, people finished work and just forgot about it until the next day! Now we are all available around the clock, which can have a damaging effect on the physical and mental well-being of staff. We're persuaded to feel guilty or even lazy if we refuse to work in our own time, but this is crazy! Eating into our 'switch-off' time harms our sleep quality, which means we can't perform efficiently during actual working hours. Some companies are beginning to appreciate that the negatives of an 'always-on' culture outweigh the positives. The German car manufacturer Volkswagen, for example, has banned email access when staff are off-shift.

Sadly, most companies aren't as enlightened as Volkswagen. A recent study of 3,000 UK business workers found that 69 per cent were regularly required to work outside their contracted hours. I see the effects of this all the time among my patients. One office manager, Warren, came in begging for sleeping pills. He told me he'd been getting around three hours' sleep a night, and even that was broken. He would toss and turn. If he couldn't sleep, he would scroll his phone in bed, check his emails or watch YouTube videos. He felt as if he had 'tried everything'. He couldn't even remember what it was like to get a good night's sleep. He had been struggling for years.

This is a common complaint. I see it all the time. But before reaching for a prescription I asked a few questions about his lifestyle. He told me he'd get into bed with his laptop and go through his work emails. It wasn't unusual for him to get agitated by the fact that one of his colleagues was sending him something at 10.30 p.m. 'It's like that guy's got it off his chest and it's now on my chest and I'm lying in bed thinking about it,' he said.

'You can't change what that guy is going to do,' I told him. 'But what can you change? You've made a decision to take the computer to bed and then you opened the email. That's a choice you make. And it really is that simple.'

'But that's my job,' he said. 'I have to check them after dinner.'

'Well, can we compromise?' I asked. 'Do you think at 8 p.m. you could switch off the laptop?'

He agreed, and that single intervention had an immediate impact. Warren began falling asleep faster and falling asleep deeper. And all this made him more amenable to further change. As he re-evaluated his relationship with his emails it also caused him to re-evaluate his relationship with his smartphone. He began allowing himself to browse social media until 9 p.m., but that was when his No-Tech 90 began. He's now sleeping seven hours per night.

Exercise, too, can count as commotion. Although a few people find that vigorous exercise in the evening doesn't affect their sleep, for many of us it can be problematic. A part of the problem is that exercise can raise cortisol levels at exactly the time of day when they should be falling. If I play a game of squash past seven o'clock I find myself lying in bed at night, my heart pounding.

Many people tell me that they cannot fall asleep unless the television is on. This is not because our television sets possess magical sleep-inducing powers, but rather because these people are go, go, go all day long. That time in front of the TV is merely the first chance they've given their body to switch off. It's not the glowing box that's causing them to fall asleep, it's the fact they're suddenly giving themselves permission to relax. Whilst chilling on the sofa in front of the television is helping them shut down, the quality of their sleep will *always* be low. My goal with these patients is to teach them a different way to switch off. They need to fall into deep, restorative sleep in the comfort of their own bed rather than on their sofa in a room filled with raised voices, police sirens, quiz-show buzzers and explosions.

To do this, I use many of the interventions in *The Four Pillar Plan*, particularly in the Sleep and Relax pillars, including making nightly entries in a gratitude journal (see page 44), which helps redirect thoughts from negativity and anxiety towards positivity and gratefulness before bed.

TIPS TO MANAGE YOUR COMMOTION

DON'T WATCH THE NEWS, A THRILLER, OR ANY SIMILAR
COMMOTION-CAUSING PROGRAMME BEFORE BED

DON'T DISCUSS FINANCIAL OR STRESSFUL
FAMILY MATTERS

MAKE IT A RULE NOT TO CHECK WORK EMAILS
IN THE NINETY MINUTES BEFORE BED

FOCUS ON RELAXING EXERCISE IN THE EVENING
SUCH AS YOGA OR LIGHT STRETCHING

TRY THE 3–4–5 BREATHING METHOD (PAGE 50)
TO HELP YOU UNWIND FROM THE DAY'S STRESSES

MEDITATION BEFORE BED CAN HELP YOU QUIETEN
YOUR MIND (SEE PAGE 47)

EDUCATE YOUR FAMILY AND FRIENDS ABOUT YOUR
EVENING ROUTINE

MAKE AN ENTRY IN YOUR GRATITUDE JOURNAL
BEFORE BED (SEE PAGE 44)

5. ENJOY YOUR CAFFEINE BEFORE NOON

Ensure that any caffeine you do choose to consume is taken before lunchtime.

Caffeine is the world's most popular drug. Millions of us love to get jacked up on the stuff on a daily basis. In the UK we drink 70 million coffees per day, which seems a lot until you discover that the number of cups of tea we down tops 165 million. And why not? Caffeine works! It helps kick-start our day and sharpens our senses, and a lot of new research associates caffeine consumption with better health outcomes. Which is lucky, because I love coffee. It's one of my life's greatest pleasures. But my passionate love affair with the dark stuff has definitely had its ups and downs. I have my own personal threshold, as you're likely to, beyond which just enough becomes too much. Drink a bit and I feel happy, energized and focused. Drink too much and I feel fatigued, shaky and anxious.

For years I convinced myself that I needed coffee to get me going. However, I began to question this when I read the results of a 2010 study from the University of Bristol suggesting that what might actually be happening is that we wake up suffering from caffeine withdrawal symptoms that make us feel terrible, and that morning cup I'm craving so badly is simply making me feel like a non-caffeine drinker does all the time. I didn't like this study, but I have to admit I think it's likely to hold true. Still, the fact remains you're going to have to prise my coffee cup out of my shaking hands! I'm not about to give it up – not just yet, anyway. In order to get most of the benefits of caffeine, and avoid many of the problems, it's about drinking the right amount at the right time.

That's going to be different for each one of us. How you metabolize coffee depends a bit on your genetics. There's a gene called the CYP1A2 that helps determine how quickly we break caffeine down. There are different variants of this gene. Some of us have a version that can break it down up to four times faster than others. If you're one of the lucky ones who metabolize it more quickly, you're also more likely to get many of caffeine's benefits, which include lower risk of stroke, Alzheimer's disease and heart attack. But if you metabolize it more slowly, it'll stick around in your body for longer and that may make you more vulnerable to its adverse effects, which include irritability, anxiety and sleep disruption.

And make no mistake about it, caffeine is a big sleep disruptor. Adenosine is a chemical that's made in the body that builds up the longer we're awake. The more adenosine we have, the more sleepy we feel. Caffeine blocks adenosine receptors. By breaking the body's ability to sense adenosine, it fools it into thinking that it's less sleepy than it really is. It's by actions such as these that caffeine can prolong sleep latency (the time it takes to fall asleep), reduce total sleep time, reduce sleep efficiency and worsen perceived sleep quality.

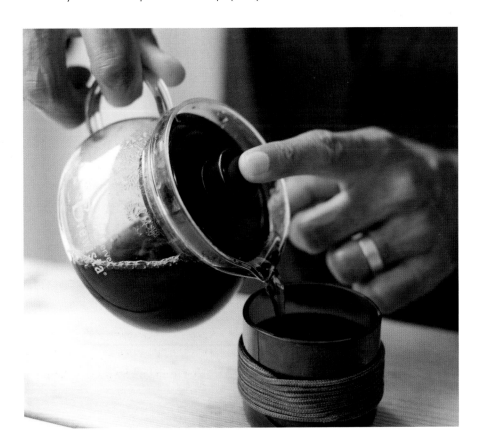

It's no surprise, then, that many people sleep a lot better when they quit caffeine completely. Some manage perfectly well by sticking to it only in the morning. The truly lucky ones can have a double espresso right before bed and drift off. I'm always amazed when I go for dinner with my wife's family, who always gleefully order powerful coffees straight after the meal. But the evidence is now suggesting that even if you can fall asleep after an evening caffeine hit, you don't access the deep levels of sleep that you need. The reality is, if you think your sleep could be better than it is, you should try to avoid caffeine after midday.

But why midday? Why not 2 p.m.? Why not 4 p.m.? All drugs have what's known as a 'half life', which is the time it takes for its initial level of effect to reduce by 50 per cent. Caffeine's half life is about six hours, although there's a bit of individual variability depending on your genetics and various lifestyle factors. That means, if you're having caffeine in the middle of the afternoon, there's a probability that it's still in your system when you're lying in bed and trying to sleep. Given that we know caffeine helps improve alertness, for many people caffeine in the afternoon will be impacting their sleep.

One of my most effective tools in helping my own sleep quality as well as that of my patients has been to implement this watershed. I've had patients who've come in demanding sleeping pills and have resisted cutting down on caffeine. They insist they've been coffee drinkers all their lives and it's never been a problem. But what if their threshold has changed? What if, when they were younger, their stress levels were lower? They might be right that caffeine didn't affect them before, but there's every chance it does now. It's not unusual for people to resist giving up caffeine after noon, especially when they remember you can also find it in many soft drinks, herbal teas and green tea, even so-called 'decaf' coffee. But when they do, it's game changing.

TIPS TO REDUCE YOUR CAFFEINE INTAKE AFTER 12 NOON

DRINK NON-CAFFEINATED HERBAL TEA TO GET YOU PAST
YOUR 3 P.M. SLUMP (REMEMBER, GREEN TEA CONTAINS CAFFEINE)

AVOID DECAFFEINATED COFFEE AS MANY
BRANDS STILL CONTAIN TRACE AMOUNTS

DRINK SPARKLING WATER IN PLACE OF YOUR
CAFFEINATED BEVERAGE

REDUCE YOUR SUGAR INTAKE (SEE PAGE 80).
THIS WILL ACTUALLY GIVE YOU MORE ENERGY AND REDUCE
THE LIKELIHOOD OF CRAVING A CAFFEINE PICK-ME-UP IN
THE AFTERNOON

DRINK CAMOMILE TEA IN THE EVENING.
THIS CAN BE A GREAT CAFFEINE REPLACEMENT
AS WELL AS PROMOTING RELAXATION BEFORE SLEEP

15 WAYS TO IMPROVE YOUR SLEEP

Why don't you start with three?

1. Take outdoor breaks in the morning

2. Enforce a strict 'no caffeine after noon' rule

3. Make a No-Tech 90 before bed a new habit

4. Set an alarm to tell you when it's time for bed

5. Fit blackout blinds in your bedroom

6. Remove ALL screens from your bedroom

7. Consider opening the bedroom window. The perfect temperature for sleeping is around 17°C/65°F

8. Eat earlier in the day, before 7 p.m. if possible

9. Exercise earlier in the day

10. Socialize earlier in the day

11. Buy red lights for night-time illumination

12. Buy amber glasses to filter blue light from screens

13. Don't use your phone as an alarm clock

14. Install f:lux on your e-devices, or switch on 'night-time mode'

15. Avoid vigorous activity in the three hours before bed

MAKING IT HAPPEN

'The mind all too often takes the path of least resistance and reverts to type. By designing our home environment we're controlling what can be controlled and maximizing our chances of success. Remember, about 90 per cent of your health is determined by your environment, not your genes.'

If you're going to implement the changes I suggest, it's critical that you design your environment for success. That means taking all the nasty industrial food products off the shelf and throwing them into the bin. It means putting your smartphone charger in your kitchen, not your bedroom. It means keeping the movement step on the floor of your kitchen so you walk past it every single day. If it's in its box, in an out-of-reach cupboard, you're never going to use it. We massively overestimate how much willpower we possess. We have finite amounts of it. There's not much you can do about the toxic environment that exists outside your front door and you'll need all the willpower you have to cope with that. The mind all too often takes the path of least resistance and reverts to type. By designing our home environment we're controlling what can be controlled and maximizing our chances of success. Remember, about 90 per cent of your health is determined by your environment, not your genes. Dr Francis Collins, director of the US National Institutes of Health, put it best when he said, 'Genes load the gun, environment pulls the trigger.'

Use this book to start changing the 90 per cent.

FINDING YOUR BALANCE

So there you have it. I have now shared with you ideas that have transformed my own life and my family's. I can honestly claim to have saved hundreds of patients from a lifetime of pain and medication. I'm pretty sure they've even saved lives. I am seeing results that it's no exaggeration to describe as near-miraculous.

I have reversed type 2 diabetes, eliminated chronic skin conditions, cured depression and made menopausal symptoms vanish. I have helped patients conquer their migraines, reduce anxiety and overcome fatigue. I now treat irritable bowel syndrome, not by suppressing its symptoms with drugs but by getting to the root cause (or causes) and eliminating them. I'm curing insomnia. I am getting rid of intractable reflux, heartburn, fatty liver, chronic back pain. I'm lowering patients' blood pressure and curing insomnia – all without the use of medication.

I share these successes, not to boast, but to show you what can be realized when you apply the principles in the book. As I said, I call this new approach 'progressive medicine'. I call it this because I'm convinced it's the direction we must go in if we want to save the NHS and save our health. There is a time and a place for medication and surgery, which can be life-saving and life-giving, but when it comes to well-being, maintaining long-term health and quality of life, the best medicine for you *is* you.

Once you learn about progressive medicine you have no choice but to embrace it. Every doctor I've told about it says the same: 'Once you know it, you can't go back.' For us in the medical establishment, progressive medicine is nothing less than an ethical obligation. It brings medicine back to its roots. One of the basic tenets of our craft is the Hippocratic oath, *primum non nocere* – first, do no harm. In our overmedicated world, this idea has gone out of the window. We need the medicine of aetiology, not symptomatology – the medicine that asks 'why' rather than simply telling you 'what'. Progressive medicine is medicine as it was always supposed to be.

Now I've passed a distillation of this knowledge to you. And now you can't unknow it. The question is, what will you do with your newfound knowledge? Behaviour change can be hard. I know this all too well. What makes *The Four Pillar Plan* different is that it is achievable for every single one of you. What job you are in doesn't matter, your ethical preference regarding food doesn't matter and where you live doesn't matter – everyone can apply its concepts in his or her own life.

As you move from two interventions to four, from four to eight and from eight to eighteen, you are building fantastically strong foundations. You're moving further beneath your threshold, becoming more resilient and more able to bounce back when life does throw you its inevitable curve balls. These small changes become your new habits and these new habits become your health. If ten minutes of meditation is too hard, start with one minute. If cutting out sugar is too daunting, start somewhere else. The key to this plan is balance – balance across all four pillars. Just as there is no One True Diet, there is no One Right Way to do this plan. Jump in and don't be afraid. Read it. Absorb it. Try it. Own it. Tell people about it. Succeed. Fail and try again. Above all, enjoy. It's a recipe for a longer, healthier and happier life. And you only have the one.

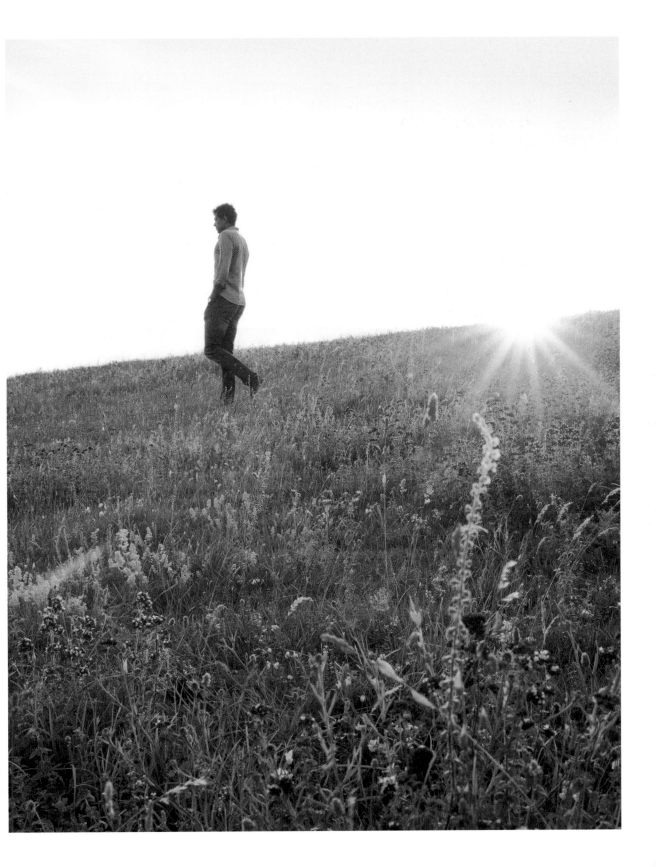

SOURCES AND FURTHER READING

RELAX

1. ME-TIME EVERY DAY

M. T. Bailey et al., 'Exposure to a Social Stressor Alters the Structure of the Intestinal Microbiota: Implications for Stressor-Induced Immunomodulation', *Brain, Behavior, and Immunity* 25(3), March 2011: 397–407, www.ncbi.nlm.nih.gov/pubmed/21040780

A. Cattaneo et al., 'Absolute Measurements of Macrophage Migration Inhibitory Factor and Interleukin-1-ß mRNA Levels Accurately Predict Treatment Response in Depressed Patients', *International Journal of Neuropsychopharmacology* 19(10), 11 May 2016: pyw045, https://academic.oup.com/ijnp/article/doi/10.1093/ijnp/pyw045/2487459/Absolute-Measurements-of-Macrophage-Migration

2. THE SCREEN-FREE SABBATH

A. Rucki, 'Average Smartphone User Checks Device 221 Times a Day, According to Research', *Evening Standard*, 7 October 2014, www.standard.co.uk/news/techandgadgets/average-smartphone-user-checks-device-221-times-a-day-according-to-research-9780810.html

D. I. Tamir and J. P. Mitchell, 'Disclosing Information About the Self is Intrinsically Rewarding', *Proceedings of the National Academy of Sciences of the United States of America* 109(21), May 2012: 8038–43, www.pnas.org/content/109/21/8038

M. Winnick, 'Putting a Finger on Our Phone Obsession', dscout, 16 June 2016, https://blog.dscout.com/mobile-touches

3. KEEP A GRATITUDE JOURNAL

C. M. Burton and L. A. King, 'The Health Benefits of Writing About Intensely Positive Experiences', *Journal of Research in Personality* 38(2), April 2004: 150–63, www.sciencedirect.com/science/article/pii/S0092656603000588

M. Popova, 'A Simple Exercise to Increase Well-Being and Lower Depression from Martin Seligman, Founding Father of Positive Psychology' [a review of *Flourish*, by Martin Seligman], www.brainpickings.org/2014/02/18/martin-seligman-gratitude-visit-three-blessings/

A. M. Wood, 'Gratitude influences sleep through the mechanism of pre-sleep cognitions', *Journal of Psychosomatic Research* 66(1) January 2009: 43–8, www.ncbi.nlm.nih.gov/pubmed/19073292

4. PRACTISE STILLNESS DAILY

Bailey et al., 'Exposure to a Social Stressor Alters the Structure of the Intestinal Microbiota'

M. Bond, 'Mind Gym: Putting Meditation to the Test', *New Scientist*, 5 January 2011, www.newscientist.com/article/mg20927940-200-mind-gym-putting-meditation-to-the-test/

K. Cherry, '"Flow" Can Help You Achieve Goals', www.verywell.com/what-is-flow-2794768

S. Simpson, 'Tiger's Roar, the Possible Secrets of Woods's Success', *The Best You*, 22 April 2013, http://thebestyoumagazine.co/tigers-roar-the-possible-secrets-of-woodss-success-by-dr-stephen-simpson/

P. Wiessner, 'Embers of Society: Firelight Talk Among the Ju/'hoansi Bushmen', *Proceedings of the National*

Academy of Sciences of the United States of America 111(39), 30 September 2014: 14027–35, www.pnas.org/content/111/39/14027

5. RECLAIM YOUR DINING TABLE

E. Robinson et al., 'Eating Attentively: A Systematic Review and Meta-Analysis of the Effect of Food Intake Memory and Awareness on Eating', *American Journal of Clinical Nutrition* 97(4), April 2013: 728–42, http://ajcn.nutrition.org/content/97/4/728.abstract

EAT

1. DE-NORMALIZE SUGAR

Diabetes UK, 'Diabetes Facts and Stats, October 2016', www.diabetes.org.uk/Documents/Position-statements/DiabetesUK_Facts_Stats_Oct16.pdf

B. S. Lennerz et al., 'Effects of Dietary Glycemic Index on Brain Regions Related to Reward and Craving in Men', *American Journal of Clinical Nutrition* 98(3), September 2013: 641–7, http://ajcn.nutrition.org/content/98/3/641

D. E. Lieberman, 'Evolution's Sweet Tooth', *The New York Times*, 5 June 2012, www.nytimes.com/2012/06/06/opinion/evolutions-sweet-tooth.html

P. M. Wise et al., 'Reduced Dietary Intake of Simple Sugars Alters Perceived Sweet Taste Intensity But Not Perceived Pleasantness', *American Journal of Clinical Nutrition* 103(1), January 2016: 50–60, www.ncbi.nlm.nih.gov/pubmed/26607941

2. A NEW DEFINITION OF 'FIVE A DAY'

J. Rosner, 'Ten Times More Microbial Cells Than Body Cells in Humans?', *Microbe* 9(2), February 2014: 47, www.researchgate.net/publication/270690292_Ten_Times_More_Microbial_Cells_than_Body_Cells_in_Humans

E. D. and J. L. Sonnenburg, 'Starving Our Microbial Self: The Deleterious Consequences of a Diet Deficient in Microbiota-Accessible Carbohydrates', *Cell Metabolism* 20(5), November 2014: 779–86, www.ncbi.nlm.nih.gov/pubmed/25156449

L. Mayer, 'Mucosal Immunity', *Pediatrics* 111, 2003: 1595–1600, www.ncbi.nlm.nih.gov/pubmed/12777598

3. INTRODUCE DAILY MICRO-FASTS

D. E. Bredesen et al., 'Reversal of Cognitive Decline in Alzheimer's Disease', *Aging* 8(6), June 2016: 1250–58, www.aging-us.com/article/100981

G. Hoeke et al., 'Role of Brown Fat in Lipoprotein Metabolism and Atherosclerosis', *Circulation Research* 118(1), January 2016: 173–83, www.ncbi.nlm.nih.gov/pubmed/26837747

Obesity Society, 'Eating Dinner Early, or Skipping It, May be Effective in Fighting Body Fat', *Science Daily*, 3 November 2016, www.sciencedaily.com/releases/2016/11/161103091229.htm

T. Tuomi et al., 'Increased Melatonin Signaling is a Risk Factor for Type 2 Diabetes', *Cell Metabolism* 23(6), June 2016: 1067–77, https://www.ncbi.nlm.nih.gov/pubmed/27185156

4. DRINK MORE WATER

H. Valtin, '"Drink at Least Eight Glasses of Water a Day" – Really? Is There Scientific Evidence for "8 X 8"?', Research Paper, Dartmouth Medical School, Lebanon, NH, August 2002, http://ajpregu.physiology.org/content/ajpregu/early/2002/08/08/ajpregu.00365.2002.full.pdf

5. UNPROCESS YOUR DIET

M. Berk et al., 'So Depression is an Inflammatory Disease, But Where Does the Inflammation Come From?', *BMC Medicine* 11, 2013: 200, www.ncbi.nlm.nih.gov/pmc/articles/PMC3846682/

S. J. Guyenet and M. W. Schwartz, 'Regulation of Food Intake, Energy Balance, and Body Fat Mass: Implications for the Pathogenesis and Treatment of Obesity', *Journal of Clinical Endocrinology & Metabolism* 97(3), March 2012: 745–55, www.ncbi.nlm.nih.gov/pmc/articles/PMC3319208/

A. R. Lubis et al., 'The Role of SOCS-3 Protein in Leptin Resistance and Obesity', *Acta Medica Indonesiana* 40(2), April 2008: 89–95, www.ncbi.nlm.nih.gov/pubmed/18560028

C. A. Monteiro et al., 'The UN Decade of Nutrition, the NOVA Food Classification and the Trouble with Ultra-Processing', *Public Health Nutrition*, 21 March 2016, https://doi.org/10.1017/S1368980017000234

I. Spreadbury, 'Comparison with Ancestral Diets Suggests Dense Acellular Carbohydrates Promote an Inflammatory Microbiota, and May be the Primary Dietary Cause of Leptin Resistance and Obesity', *Diabetes, Metabolic Syndrome and Obesity* 5, 2012: 175–89, www.ncbi.nlm.nih.gov/pmc/articles/PMC3402009/

MOVE

World Health Organization, 'Physical Inactivity: A Global Public Health Problem', www.who.int/dietphysicalactivity/factsheet_inactivity/en/

S. Daniells, 'US Army Exploring How Stressors Affect Gut Health in Soldiers: US Army Study on Extreme Exercise', NUTRA ingredients-USA.com, 20 April 2017, www.nutraingredients-usa.com/Research/US-Army-exploring-how-stressors-affect-gut-health-in-soldiers

E. Denou et al., 'High-Intensity Exercise Training Increases the Diversity and Metabolic Capacity of the Mouse Distal Gut Microbiota During Diet-Induced Obesity', *American Journal of Physiology – Endocrinology and Metabolism* 310(11), April 2016: E982–3, www.ncbi.nlm.nih.gov/labs/articles/27117007/

N. Owen et al., 'Sedentary Behavior: Emerging Evidence for a New Health Risk', *Mayo Clinic Proceedings* 85(12), December 2010: 1138–41, www.ncbi.nlm.nih.gov/pmc/articles/PMC2996155/

C. Szoeke et al., 'Predictive Factors for Verbal Memory Performance Over Decades of Aging: Data from the Women's Healthy Ageing Project', *American Journal of Geriatric Psychiatry* 24(10), October 2016: 857–67, www.ajgponline.org/article/S1064-7481(16)30113-0/abstract

1. WALK MORE

K. Berra et al., 'Making Physical Activity Counseling a Priority in Clinical Practice: The Time for Action is Now', *Journal of the American Medical Association* 314(24), December 2015: 2617–18, http://jamanetwork.com/journals/jama/article-abstract/2475164

K. J. Reid et al., 'Timing and Intensity of Light Correlate with Body Weight in Adults', *PLoS One*, 2 April 2014, http://journals.plos.org/plosone/article?id=10.1371/journal.pone.0092251

P. Srikanthan and A. S. Karlamangla, 'Muscle Mass Index as Predictor of Longevity', *American Journal of Medicine* 127(6), June 2014: 547–53, www.ncbi.nlm.nih.gov/pmc/articles/PMC4035379/

World Health Organization, Global Health Risks: Mortality and Burden of Disease Attributable to Selected Major Risks (Geneva: World Health Organization, 2009)

2. BECOME STRONGER

S. T. Arthur and I. D. Cooley, 'The Effect of Physiological Stimuli on Sarcopenia; Impact of Notch and Wnt Signaling on Impaired Aged Skeletal Muscle Repair', *International Journal of Biological Sciences* 8(5), May 2012: 731–60, www.ncbi.nlm.nih.gov/pmc/articles/PMC3371570

D. D. Cohen et al., 'Ten-Year Secular Changes in Muscular Fitness in English Children', *Acta Paediatrica* 100(10), October 2011: e175–7, https://www.ncbi.nlm.nih.gov/pubmed/21480987

Harvard Health Publications, 'Give Grip Strength a Hand', November 2016, www.health.harvard.edu/healthy-aging/give-grip-strength-a-hand

T. Liu-Ambrose et al., 'Resistance Training and Executive Functions: A 12-Month Randomized Controlled Trial', *Archives of Internal Medicine* 170(2), 2010: 170–78, http://jamanetwork.com/journals/jamainternalmedicine/article-abstract/415534

3. BEGIN REGULAR HIGH-INTENSITY INTERVAL TRAINING

J. B. Gillen et al., 'Twelve Weeks of Sprint Interval Training Improves Indices of Cardiometabolic Health Similar to Traditional Endurance Training Despite a Five-Fold Lower Exercise Volume and Time Commitment', *PLoS One*, 26 April 2016, http://journals.plos.org/plosone/article?id=10.1371/journal.pone.0154075

A. T. Piepmeier and J. L. Etnier, 'Brain-Derived Neurotrophic Factor (BDNF) as a Potential Mechanism of the Effects of Acute Exercise on Cognitive Performance', *Journal of Sport and Health Science* 4(1), March 2015: 14–23, www.sciencedirect.com/science/article/pii/S2095254614001161

M. M. Robinson et al., 'Enhanced Protein Translation Underlies Improved Metabolic and Physical Adaptations to Different Exercise Training Modes in Young and Old Humans', *Cell Metabolism* 25(3), March 2017: 581–92, www.cell.com/cell-metabolism/pdfExtended/S1550-4131(17)30099-2

B. Winter et al., 'High Impact Running Improves Learning', *Neurobiology of Learning and Memory* 87(4), May 2007: 597–609, www.ncbi.nlm.nih.gov/pubmed/17185007

SLEEP

D. Dawson and K. Reid, 'Fatigue, Alcohol and Performance Impairment' *Nature*, 17 July 1997,www.nature.com/nature/journal/v388/n6639/abs/388235a0.html

Guang Yang et al., 'Sleep Promotes Branch-Specific Formation of Dendritic Spines After Learning', *Science* 344(6188), June 2014: 1173–8, http://science.sciencemag.org/content/344/6188/1173

Lulu Xie et al., 'Sleep Drives Metabolite Clearance from the Adult Brain', *Science* 342(6156), October 2013: 373–7, http://science.sciencemag.org/content/342/6156/373

V. A. Poroyko et al., 'Chronic Sleep Disruption Alters Gut Microbiota, Induces Systemic and Adipose Tissue Inflammation and Insulin Resistance in Mice', *Nature Scientific Reports* 6, 2016, www.nature.com/articles/srep35405

2. EMBRACE MORNING LIGHT

P. G. Lindqvist et al., 'Avoidance of Sun Exposure as a Risk Factor for Major Causes of Death: A Competing Risk Analysis of the Melanoma in Southern Sweden Cohort', *Journal of International Medicine* 280(4), October 2016: 375–87, http://onlinelibrary.wiley.com/doi/10.1111/joim.12496/abstract

Poroyko et al., 'Chronic Sleep Disruption Alters Gut Microbiota'

Reid et al., 'Timing and Intensity of Light Correlate with Body Weight in Adults'

3. CREATE A BEDTIME ROUTINE

A. J. K. Phillips, 'Irregular Sleep/Wake Patterns are Associated with Poorer Academic Performance and Delayed Circadian and Sleep/Wake Timing', *Nature Scientific Reports* 7, 2017, www.nature.com/articles/s41598-017-03171-4

M. Smolensky and L. Lamberg, *The Body Clock Guide to Better Health* (New York: Henry Holt, 2001)

R. Zhang, 'A Circadian Gene Expression Atlas in Mammals: Implications for Biology and Medicine', *Proceedings of the National Academy of Sciences of the United States of America* 11(45), November 2014: 16219–24, www.pnas.org/content/111/45/16219.abstract

4. MANAGE YOUR COMMOTION

BBC News, 'Volkswagen Turns Off Blackberry Email After Work Hours', 8 March 2012, www.bbc.co.uk/news/technology-16314901

5. ENJOY YOUR CAFFEINE BEFORE NOON

V. Březinová, 'Effect of Caffeine on Sleep: EEG Study in Late Middle Age People', *British Journal of Clinical Pharmacology* 1(3), June 1974: 203–8, www.ncbi.nlm.nih.gov/pmc/articles/PMC1402564

I. Clark et al., 'Coffee, Caffeine, and Sleep: A Systematic Review of Epidemiological Studies and Randomized Controlled Trials', *Sleep Medicine Reviews* 31, January 2016: 70–78, www.ncbi.nlm.nih.gov/labs/articles/26899133

C. Drake et al., 'Caffeine Effects on Sleep Taken 0, 3, or 6 Hours Before Going to Bed', *Journal of Clinical Sleep Medicine* 9(11), November 2013: 1195–1200, www.ncbi.nlm.nih.gov/pubmed/24235903

P. J. Rogers et al., 'Association of the Anxiogenic and Alerting Effects of Caffeine with ADORA2A and ADORA1 Polymorphisms and Habitual Level of Caffeine Consumption', *Neuropsychopharmacology* 35, June 2010: 1973–83 (2010 University of Bristol study into whether there are any real benefits to habitual coffee consumption), www.nature.com/npp/journal/v35/n9/full/npp201071a.html

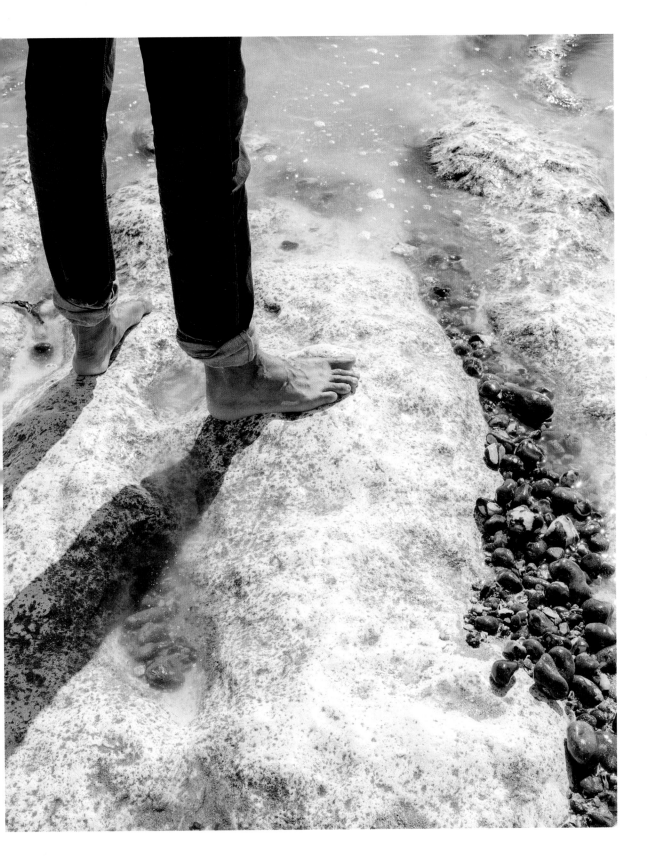

ACKNOWLEDGEMENTS

It would have been impossible to complete this project without the help and support of many incredible people. If I have missed someone out from the list below, my deepest apologies – it was unintentional.

Dad, so much has happened since you have gone that I know would have made you immensely proud. As I grow into fatherhood, I appreciate what you did with so much more clarity and understanding. Thank you.

Mum, you have been the driving force behind me since the day I was born. You always pushed me to be the best that I can be and have selflessly given me everything I could have ever wanted. Thank you for your unwavering support, unconditional love and always believing. You have taught me about compassion and how to care.

Vidhaata, you are my rock. You have un-fogged the misty glasses through which I used to view life. Your love, honesty and ability to look deep inside my soul have changed me for the better. You have given me confidence and helped me cultivate the ability to truly be myself. This will be a long and winding road but it's going to be a lot of fun and we have only just begun.

For my children, I am in awe of the lessons that you teach me every single day. You have shown me the beautiful simplicity in being present and happy. Thank you for keeping meticulous track of my word count and reminding me what is truly important in life. I hope this book makes you proud and helps create a happier, healthier world for you to grow up in.

Dada, I am lucky to have never known life without you. You are the most caring and supportive big brother anyone could ever wish for. I can rely on you for absolutely anything and that means so much to me. You are *always* there, no matter what I need, no matter what time. You make me incredibly proud.

Chetana and Dinesh – I am fortunate to have gained a new set of parents – you have welcomed me in as one of your own. Thanks for the love, friendship and support you provide to me, and the entire family.

Ayan – you are like a brother to me. Thanks for being 'on-call' day in, day out. This journey is made much easier, and much more fun, with your brotherly arm around me. Reconnecting with you has been a joy.

Jeremy – thank you for being a trusted voice whether it be for advice, work or just a bit of fun. I am lucky to call you a friend.

Mike – words will never be able to thank you enough. Your generosity, ongoing support, mentorship as well as multiple proofreads would be more than enough but, most of all, thank you for your friendship.

Luke – for being yourself, the creative input and the proofreading. You are a true friend.

Steve, Karron and Ashley – for unconditional friendship and support.

Antony – for the connection.

James Maskell – you have always helped me get the word out there and I am honoured to have you as a close friend and ally.

Gary – for fixing my back and contributing to this book. It was a fun process that I know will help so many.

Al – for your generosity and honesty.

To Will Francis and Will Storr – for the creative input and the camaraderie.

Special thanks to Bobby Chatterjee, Philip McCabe, Daniel Bryson, Jodie Hawkey, Mary Salama, Phil Creswell, Mark Warnes, Sarbani, Clare Moore, Claire Gardin, Aidan Tarran-Jones, James Acton, Dhru Purohit, Dallas Hartwig, Kelly Brogan, Mark Hyman, Darryl Edwards, Christian Platt, Charles Poliquin, Satchinanda Panda, Dale Bredesen, Bernice Hulme, Sophie Laurimore and the Factual team.

To John and Susan – thank you for helping bring my vision to life.

Thank you to the whole team at Penguin Life who have believed in me and supported me throughout. In particular, Venetia, Emily, Sarah, Emma, Julia, Isabel, and Josie.

Lastly, to all of my patients, you have taught me more than I could ever have learned myself – thank you.

INDEX

A

acellular carbohydrates 136, 138

adenosine 245

ageing

> and high-intensity interval training 174

> and strength training 161, 164–5

Akkermansia muciniphila 98, 110

anti-inflammatory diet 133, 136–9

aryl hydrocarbon receptor (AHR) 96

Attenborough, David 70

autonomic nervous system 25

autophagy 108–9, 205

B

bedtime routine 232–7

berries 103

blue light 216, 219

blue-zone diets 76

body clock 112–13, 159

> bedtime routine 232–7

> suprachiasmatic nucleus 214

brain derived neurotrophic factor (BDNF) 175

breathing exercises 50–59, 65, 243

Bredesen, Dale 109

Burton, Chad 45

C

Cacioppo, John 68

caffeine 244–7

carbohydrates 126, 127, 136–7

cellular carbohydrates 136–7

circadian rhythm 112–13, 159

> bedtime routine 232–7

> suprachiasmatic nucleus 214

coffee 244–7

Collins, Francis 250

commotion 238–43

computers 234, 235, 241–2

> see also smartphones; tablets

cortisol steal 26–7

cortisol surge 22–4

Crohn's disease 30–32

cytokines 32, 160

D

dairy 78–9

darkness 213–20

depression, and inflammation 28–9, 132

diabetes 81, 84–5, 86

    and sleep 208–9, 210

diet *see* Eat

digestive system

    leaky gut 128

    and stress 27

digital detox 36–43

dining table 66–71

E

Eat 14, 74–9

    de-normalizing sugar 80–89

    drink more water 119–23

    introduce daily micro-fasts 108–114

    a new definition of 'five a day'
    90–107

    unprocess your diet 124–48

Edwards, Darryl 179

emotional commotion 238–43

exercise *see* Move

extensor chain muscles 184–6

F

fasting 98, 108–114

fats 126–7, 138–9

fibre 98, 132

firelight talk 68

five a day 90–107

five-minute kitchen workout 165, 166–7,
    179

flex on a step 190–91

flexor chain muscles 184

flow 62–3

food *see* Eat

foot clocks 194–5

Foster, Russell 215

The Four Pillar Plan 14–15, 250–52

 Eat 73–145

 Move 147–98

 Relax 17–71

 Sleep 201–249

G

ghrelin 208

Gibala, Martin 174

gluten 78–9

glutes 182–98

glycosinolates 100

grains 78–9

gratitude journal 44–7, 242, 243

gut 30–32

 leaky gut 128, 130, 151, 209

 microbiome 49–50, 90–98, 155

H

high-intensity interval training (HIIT) 160, 170–77

hip adduction 192–3

hip extension 196–7

I

Ikaria 237

immune system

 cytokines 32

 and fasting 110

 and microbiome 93, 94–7

 and movement 155

 and sleep deprivation 208

 and stress 28–9

inflammation 28–9, 94, 132

 anti-inflammatory diet 133

 and fasting 110

 and LPS 130

 and mitochondria 111

 and movement 160, 174

 and polyphenols 139

 and sleep 209

insulin 84, 86, 174

insulin receptors 160

insulin resistance 85, 86, 209

interleukin 6, 32, 160

intestinal permeability 128

J

Ju/'hoansi bushmen 68

K

kitchen workout 165, 166–7, 179

L

lactose intolerance 78–9

LDL cholesterol 26

leaky gut 128, 130, 151, 209

leptin 134–6, 208, 209

Levine, James 152

Lieberman, Daniel 82

light 214–15, 219

    blue light 216, 219

    morning light 159, 222–30

    red light 218, 219

lipopolysaccharides (LPS) 130

loneliness 68

Louden, Andrew 112–13

low-carb diets 126, 127

low-fat diets 126–7

M

me-time every day 22–35

meditation 47–50, 60, 65, 243

menopause 30

micro-fasts 108–114

microbiome 49–50, 90–98, 132

    and movement 155

microbiota-accessible carbohydrates (MACs) 98

microsleeps 237

mindfulness 48–9, 60

mitochondria 110, 111

    and movement 155, 160, 174

mobile phones *see* smartphones

morning light 159, 222–30

Move 15, 148–55

    become stronger 160–69

    high-intensity interval training 170–77

    movement snacking 178–81

    wake up your sleepy glutes 182–98

    walk more 156–9

muscle 160–62

    see also glutes

N

naps 237

nature 226–8

nervous system 25

No-Tech 90, 234, 235, 243

O

office workout 180

Ohsumi, Yoshinori 108

Okinawa 126, 127

Oliver, Jamie 234

P

Panda, Satchidananda 109

parasympathetic nervous system 25, 70

perfectionist presentation 40

phones *see* smartphones

physical activity *see* Move

phytonutrients 100–103, 104–7

    polyphenols 100, 102–3, 139

Poliquin, Charles 44, 119

polyphenols 100, 102–3, 139

Poulain, Michel 76

Primal Play Tag 179

Primal Play Tag 179

processed foods 124, 126–7, 132, 140–42

progressive medicine 8–12, 251–2

protein 88, 143, 145

R

RATE chart 210–211

real food 142–5

Rechtschaffen, Allan 204

red light 218, 219, 235

Relax 14, 18, 20

    keep a gratitude journal 44–7

    me-time every day 22–35

    practise stillness daily 47–65

    reclaim your dining table 66–71

    screen-free Sabbath 36–43

S

sarcopenia 161, 164–5

Seligman, Martin 45

serotonin 227

Shaw, George Bernard 178

short-chain fatty acids (SCFAs) 94, 98

sitting 152–4

Sleep 15, 202–211, 248–9

    create a bedtime routine 232–7

    create an environment of absolute darkness 213–20

    enjoy your caffeine before noon 244–7

    manage your commotion 238–43

smartphones

    addiction 38–40

    reset your relationship 40–42

    seven-day digital detox 42–3

    and sleep 216, 219, 234, 235

snacks 88, 104, 139

social connection 68

social media 36–40

Spreadbury, Ian 136–7

stillness 47–65

strength training 160–69

stress 132

    and autonomic nervous system 25

    cortisol steal 26–7

    cortisol surge 23–4

    and digestive system 27

    and the gut 30–32, 49–50

    and immune system 28–9

    and the menopause 30

    and sleep deprivation 208

sugar 80–81

    changing your taste buds 81–2

    and diabetes 84–6

    strategies with craving 89

    strategies to cut down 88

    symptoms of overreliance 83

    taking the plunge 87

sun salutation 63

Sundays, screen-free Sabbath 36–43

sunlight 222–30

suprachiasmatic nucleus (SCN) 214

Surya Namaskar 63

sympathetic nervous system 25

T

television 217, 243

3-4-5 breathing 50–59, 65, 243

3D hip extension 196–7

W

water 119–23

RELAX

NOTES

_____

_____

_____

_____

_____

_____

_____

_____

_____

_____

_____

_____

_____

_____

_____

_____

_____

_____

_____

EAT

NOTES

_____

_____

_____

_____

_____

_____

_____

_____

_____

_____

_____

_____

_____

_____

_____

_____

_____

MOVE

NOTES

SLEEP

NOTES

_____

_____

_____

_____

_____

_____

_____

_____

_____

_____

_____

_____

_____

_____

_____

_____

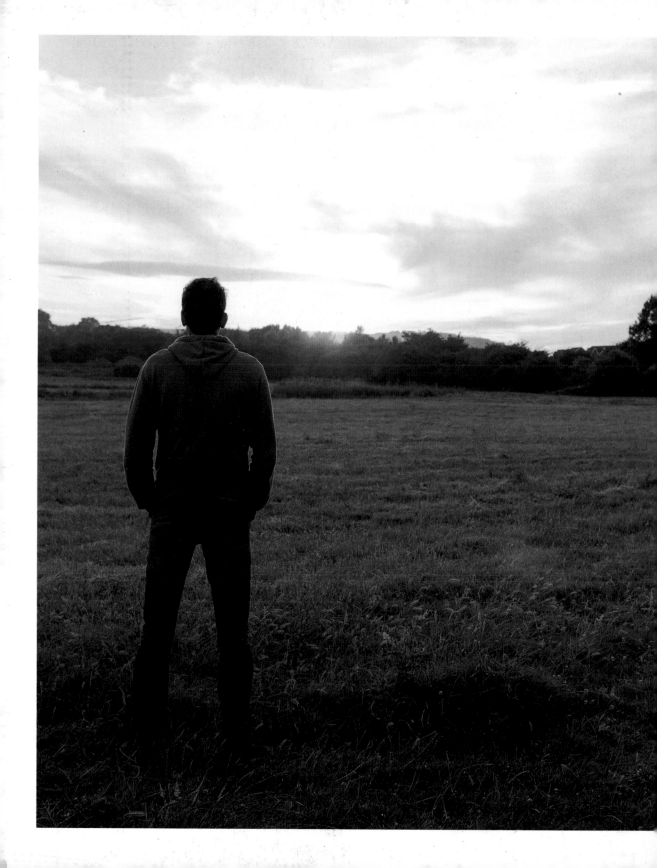